This book would not have been possible without the support of Richard and Paul.

Thank you.

For Churchill Livingstone

Commissioning Editor: Ellen Green; Jacqueline Curthoys
Project Editor: Mairi McCubbin
Design Direction: Judith Wright

Nursing and Politics
Power through Practice

Edited by
Abigail Masterson MN BSc RN PGCEA

Director, Abi Masterson Consulting Ltd, UK

Sian Maslin-Prothero MSc DipN(Lond) CertEd RN RM

Lecturer in Nursing, University of Nottingham, UK

Foreword by
Ann Keen RN DN PGCEA (District Nursing)

MP for Brentford and Isleworth

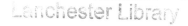
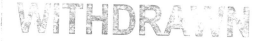
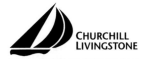
CHURCHILL
LIVINGSTONE

EDINBURGH LONDON NEW YORK PHILADELPHIA SYDNEY TORONTO 1999

CHURCHILL LIVINGSTONE
An imprint of Harcourt Brace and Company Limited

© Harcourt Brace and Company Limited 1999

⚓ is a registered trade mark of Harcourt Brace and
Company Limited 1999

First published 1999
ISBN 0 443 059918

British Library Cataloguing in Publication Data
A catalogue record for this book is available from the British
Library.

Library of Congress Cataloging in Publication Data
A catalog record for this book is available from the Library of
Congress.

The
publisher's
policy is to use
**paper manufactured
from sustainable forests**

Printed in China
EPC/01

Contents

Contributors

Ailsa Cameron BA MSc
Research Fellow, School for Policy Studies, University of Bristol, Bristol

4 The role of interest groups

John Dearlove BSc(Econ) MA DPhil
Dean of the School of Social Sciences, University of Sussex, Brighton

3 The role of political parties

Elaine Denny BSc MA CertEd RGN RHV
Senior Lecturer, School of Health and Policy Studies, University of Central England, Birmingham

1 The politics of health

Linda East BSc MPhil RGN
Lecturer in Nursing Studies, University of Nottingham, Queen's Medical Centre, Nottingham

5 The role of local government

Sian Maslin-Prothero MSc DipN(Lond) CertEd RN RM
Lecturer in Nursing, University of Nottingham, Queen's Medical Centre, Nottingham

7 Power, politics and nursing

Abigail Masterson MN BSc RGN PGCEA
Director, Abi Musterson Consulting Ltd, Bristol

7 *Power, politics and nursing*

Jean S. Neave BA(Hons) MSc RGN RHV
Formerly Principal Lecturer, Applied Behavioural Studies, Thames Valley University, London

6 *Parliament, UK politics and the European Union*

Elizabeth Perkins BSc(Hons) PhD RGN
Director, Health and Community Care Research Unit, University of Liverpool, Liverpool

2 *An introduction to political concepts*

Paul Taggart BA MA MPhil PhD
Lecturer in Politics, School of Social Sciences, University of Sussex, Brighton

3 *The role of political parties*

Foreword

For too long nurses have been on the fringes of national politics. On the 1st May 1997 however, Laura Moffat (Lab, Crawley) and I became the first two nurses elected to Parliament.

We now have a government that has appointed the first Public Health Minister, acknowledged the direct link between poverty and ill-health, and has begun to address the gross inequalities that exist in the provision of health care. Nurses must be encouraged to be political at every level of politics. This is necessary for the future of the nursing profession and equitable care provision for patients. There are many opportunities on offer, but many more to be created.

The election of Laura and I was timely, reflecting an increase in responsibilities for nurses within the NHS. For example the changing nature of health care provision, nurse prescribing, and the change of emphasis out of the hospital and into the community will greatly increase the profile of nurses – especially community nurses.

We must embrace the opportunities available to us, take on the new statutory leadership role for nurses in Primary Care Groups, and make ourselves heard. Nurse education and leadership must encourage this to take place. I hope that, through stimulating interest and awareness in the political process, this book will also motivate nurses to make their voices heard.

1998   A. K.

Preface

British politics has been undergoing dramatic and fundamental change. As the country's economy languished in recession new patterns of political alignment, new types of political organization and new sources of political conflict emerged. In 1973 the United Kingdom (UK) joined the European Community (EC) and ceded certain crucial powers to the European bureaucracy in Brussels. Governments, both in the UK and the European Union (EU), rarely give nurses or nursing more than a passing mention. Nurses have faced constant difficulties in trying to place their work on the political agenda. Yet knowledge of the political system is vital if nurses are to be effective in influencing policy and the allocation of resources.

Many nurses are uncomfortable with the idea of politics, seeing it as an undesirable distraction from their core purpose of care delivery, but politics impact on every aspect of nursing at both macro and micro levels. There has been no academic politics text specifically aimed at nurses in the last 10 years, despite repeated calls within the profession for nurses to 'get political'. The International Council for Nurses has declared that one of its key objectives is to strengthen the profile of nursing associations and improve nurses' political expertise. The Council justifies this goal by saying that nurses need to recognize that many of the daily dilemmas and choices they face are imposed on them because of decisions taken elsewhere. In part as a result of such lobbying by professional organizations, the subject of politics is now a core component of many pre- and post-registration courses. We, the editors, have considerable experience in teaching politics to nurses and this book is a synthesis of that experience. Unlike the majority of generic politics texts, which seldom mention nursing, this book takes a particular nursing focus, both in its content and in its analysis.

Neither we nor our contributors are exclusively committed to any one theory or viewpoint. Politics is a complicated discipline and it makes no sense, in an introductory text, to portray all wisdom as residing in one perspective. The study of politics entails the analysis of power in all its aspects. To achieve this we believe that it is necessary to consider critically the insights that derive from a number of rival traditions. This book is deliberately aimed at creating debate and stimulating awareness rather than providing answers.

We are convinced that when nurses become familiar with the ways in which power and politics are interlinked, and with their impact on patterns and processes of care, they will begin to feel more able to participate in policy and decision-making processes at all levels. The aim of this book is to stimulate such interest and awareness. The book is aimed at nurses, midwives and health visitors in every area of practice and will be of particular interest to those studying politics and policy making in pre- and post-registration education. However, it will also be of general interest to other health and social care professionals.

At the end of each chapter there are references, suggested further reading and key questions for personal reflection and discussion. These have been designed to enable you to see the relevance and meaning of the ideas to you as an individual and to your practice as a nurse. We hope that you will progressively internalize the concepts and theories discussed to the extent that they will permeate your practice.

THE PLAN OF THE BOOK

Elaine Denny opens the discussion in Chapter 1 by introducing you to the ideas contained in the politics of health. She explains that latterly there has been an explicit reconsideration of the idea of health need and a greater emphasis on setting priorities in the delivery of health care. She goes on to chronicle the recent reappraisal of the Welfare State and the widespread loss of faith in traditional approaches to welfare production and distribution. The introduction and development of an 'internal market' is examined as a mechanism designed to result in more efficient services, increased accountability in service delivery and improved outcomes. Denny highlights that, although nurses occupy positions on both sides of the internal market, the nursing perspective is frequently absent from wider political debates about health care planning and provision, both nationally and internationally.

In Chapter 2 Elizabeth Perkins explores political concepts and perspectives such as capitalism, Marxism, labourism, liberalism, New Right, conservatism, feminism and race. These theoretical foundations are shown to be essential if nurses are to understand fully the complexities of political analysis. Perkins also builds on the book's main theme of the importance and relevance to nurses of the study and understanding of politics.

In Chapter 3 Paul Taggart and John Dearlove review the role of political parties in modern representative democracies. Political parties have long been seen as enhancing democracy and encouraging the efficient discharge of public affairs by some political commentators. The Labour and Conservative parties are in decline in terms of their capacity to attract votes and new members, and to respond to new issues. The fact that the Conservatives were able to hold on to power for nearly 2 decades raises questions about the concept of democracy in new Britain. Women and minority ethnic groups (amongst others) have cause to criticize the limited extent of their representation in political parties, Parliament and government. Each of the two main parties has a somewhat different attitude to health policy. Historically, at least, parties on the political left have spent more on redistributive and ameliorative services in both local and central government; however, New Labour poses a serious challenge to this assumption. Third parties continue to be unable to turn votes into seats. Electoral reform could go some way towards making the system more representative, but there are limits as to what this would achieve, particularly if the parties themselves are less than representative and democratic in the ways in which they organize their own affairs. Nurses have little impact at parliamentary level, although they are making a contribution at local government level. This chapter aims to make sense of nursing's political potential against a backdrop of election manifestos and contemporary policies.

Ailsa Cameron considers the role of interest groups in politics and policy making in Chapter 4. Nursing and professions allied to medicine are used as case studies to illustrate the function of interest groups in the political process. Interest groups articulate a single interest or policy and exert pressure on governments in the hope of shaping a facet of public policy to their advantage. The analytical perspectives outlined in Chapter 2 are built on to offer a variety of explanations of the importance of interest groups generally. For example, pluralists see many groups as influential, Marxists attend to the power of business, New Right theorists advocate the importance of trade unions and sectional groups, feminists are concerned with the power of male groups and black theorists argue that the world is biased in favour of white interests. The interests of minority groups also include gay men and women and minority ethnic groups. All of these perspectives are considered in the context of the case studies.

Linda East explores the role of local government in Chapter 5, and examines the changing role of local government in relation to nursing and the provision of health and social services. The system of local government warrants particular attention because local government is elected, provides a variety of services, accounts for a quarter of public expenditure and raises some of its own revenue through the council tax. The development of competitive tendering forced competition with the independent and voluntary sectors to provide services for people with disabilities and older people. Changes in the funding and organization of continuing care and its impact on nurses working with older people will act as focal point for the analysis.

Jean Neave, in Chapter 6, takes us through the role of Parliament, UK politics and the European Union. Law is a crucial arena for political struggle because politics often revolves around the claim for rights, and much statute law made by Parliament is developed in response to organized pressures. An analysis of health care and nursing statutes and statutory instruments adds richness to the discussion. Neave emphasizes why an understanding of Parliament's function is necessary to make sense of the current situation and role of nursing in UK politics. Entry into the European Community in 1973 challenged parliamentary sovereignty and Britain's capacity to govern itself through a democratically elected Parliament. In crucial areas of health and social policy Britain is affected by the EU, which actually determines what the law should be, for example, the number and type of hours of curriculum content for nursing registration. The institutions of the EU, such as the Commission, Council of Ministers, the European Parliament, the European Council, the Court of Justice and others, are examined and their implications for UK health policy and nursing practice outlined.

The politics of nursing is the concern of Chapter 7, the final chapter, in which we aim to develop further the professional awareness of politics and understanding of its positive and negative impacts on the profession of nursing, the context of care and the content of practice. Through this analysis and the knowledge base existing in this text we hope to empower nurses to respond in an informed way to the changes they face and will continue to face. We believe that nurses must influence the political agenda for health in order to challenge the inequitable access to health and health care resources, economic impoverishment and unsafe physical surroundings that currently threaten the health and well-being of countless people in the UK.

As nurses we work in health care systems that exclude or disadvantage large numbers of people who need care and we are frequently confronted by health problems caused by ageism, sexism, racism and the unequal distribution of human rights. In addition, the consequences of environmental devastation threaten health on a global scale. Despite a commitment to health in nursing we tend, as professionals, to focus on patients/clients as individuals and on the minutiae of the nurse–patient relationship. We fail to challenge the institutional context or address issues such as inequality which have a damaging effect on the delivery of nursing care. Chapter 7 outlines an exciting view of the emancipative potential of nursing.

We conclude by drawing together the theoretical arguments and historical evidence reviewed in earlier chapters in an attempt to clarify the nature of the changes that affect nursing today.

1998   A. M.

                                                                                                  S. M. P.

Abbreviations

AIDS:	acquired immune deficiency syndrome
BMA:	British Medical Association
BSE:	bovine spongiform encephalopathy
CJD:	Creutzfeldt–Jakob disease
CHE:	Commission on Health and Environment
CLD:	Commission for Local Democracy
COI:	Central Office of Information
DOH:	Department of Health
DG:	Directorate-General
DSO:	Direct Service Organization
EC:	European Community
EEC:	European Economic Community
EU:	European Union
GLC:	Greater London Council
GP:	general practitioner
HIV:	human immunodeficiency virus
MP:	Member of Parliament
NHS:	National Health Service
NVQ:	National Vocational Qualification
QUANGO:	quasi-autonomous non-governmental organization
RCN:	Royal College of Nursing
SDP:	Social Democratic Party
TGWU:	Transport and General Workers' Union
UKCC:	United Kingdom Central Council (for Nursing, Midwifery, and Health Visiting)
WHO:	World Health Organization

The politics of health

Elaine Denny

INTRODUCTION

At the inception of the National Health Service (NHS) in 1948 it was accepted that the state should be the major provider of welfare, and that the main function of a health service was to treat the sick. There were clear ideas about 'health' and 'illness', and the distinction between them. Patients were passive recipients of services planned and provided by a paternalistic, provider driven service. Now, nearly 50 years later, these ideas appear rather simplistic and dated. The boundary between health and ill health has become increasingly blurred. People live independent and active lives with varying degrees of illness and disability. Quality of life has emerged as a major consideration and health is no longer viewed as being merely absence of disease.

Throughout the 1980s and 1990s people have been encouraged by both government and health professionals to take more responsibility for their own health through adopting a healthy lifestyle. Health problems have been seen increasingly as a consequence of factors under the individual's control. Consumer involvement in services is growing and individuals and groups are demanding more say in their own health and health care.

There has been a blurring of the distinction between private and public provision of services. The private and voluntary sectors have, through central government incentives, been encouraged to expand and create alternative sources of health and social care provision. Issues of health and health care that were viewed as straightforward and unproblematic in 1948 are now perceived to be complex and multifactoral.

This chapter will consider some of the pressures on both the supply of and demand for health care which have been influential in changing the way health services are funded and provided. I will begin by looking at the development of welfare provision in the UK and will explain how the prevailing political ideology influenced the shape it took. The postwar political consensus on welfare will be outlined in the context of the NHS and the reasons for its breakdown explored. Changing concepts of health and the complex power relationship between providers and recipients of health services will be illustrated by discussion around nursing practice issues. These practice issues include the rise of alternative or complementary medicine, explanations of the growing interest in the concept of empowerment and reasons behind the recent interest in the surveillance of the population through risk assessment.

I will conclude by speculating upon the future for the NHS, in the light of the first Labour government for 18 years.

THE HISTORICAL DEVELOPMENT OF HEALTH AND WELFARE PROVISION IN THE UK

The 19th century saw a massive growth in the provision of welfare to the poor. This growth was not, for the most part, organized by the state, but by voluntary effort. Industrialization and urbanization had led to great changes in living patterns and the separation of the workplace from the home. This is turn led to a reduction in the ability of family members to provide health care for each other.

Philanthropic and charitable associations were part of the dominant Victorian political and social culture. The free market reigned supreme and those who prospered were seen as owing an obligation to those who did not. This obligation was not open-ended, and poverty alone was not seen as an entitlement to aid. Notions of 'deserving' and 'non-deserving' were influential in deciding who should receive welfare.

State support was mainly via the Poor Law Amendment Act of 1834, which was intended as a deterrent. The doctrine of 'less eligibility' applied, whereby conditions in the poor law institutions or workhouses had to be worse than the worst conditions outside. Nevertheless, the 1834 Act did herald a recognition, albeit in a limited way, that the state had a role to play in the provision of welfare. Public health legislation, in keeping with *laissez-faire* attitudes, was enabling rather than obligatory.

This circumscribed role for the state was supported by the nation's dominant interest groups and aimed to create 'a political economy premised on a sharp distinction between the public and the private and a belief in the superiority of market outcomes and the perverse consequences of state intervention' (Cronin 1991, p. 19).

An increased role for the state in welfare provision began in liberal democracies like Sweden and the newly unified Germany at the end of the 19th century, and soon spread to other countries like Great Britain. The impetus for this change was the needs of industry rather than the needs of individuals, and consequently it was working people who were the main beneficiaries. The 1911 National Insurance Act, for example, gave limited health care benefits only to the contributor (i.e. the worker), not to other family members.

The period between 1870 and the Second World War has been described by Midwinter (1994) as one of 'creeping collectivism' (Midwinter 1994, p. 68) which was 'piecemeal and sporadic in origin and incidence' (Midwinter 1994, p. 71). In other words, the role of the state did not constitute a progressive evolution towards a particular goal, but was *ad hoc* in nature. It was increasingly recognized that the social problems associated with population growth, industrialization and urbanization had not been adequately dealt with by philanthropy and limited government intervention, and there was a growing sense that collectivist approaches would be more effective. This movement was spurred on by developments such as the expansion of suffrage, and the linking of poverty to the economic environment by early social researchers like Charles Booth (1840–1916).

In health, increasing collectivism coincided with a change in philosophy from prevention through measures such as public health legislation and the Poor Law to a curative approach. The number of hospital beds rose dramatically over this period, and for the first time 'hospital' became an acceptable place for the sick.

WELFARE PROVISION AND THE SECOND WORLD WAR

A catalyst for this major shift in ideology on the provision of welfare was undoubtedly the Second World War. In 1939 the government instituted quite Draconian powers over the conduct of people's personal lives in an unprecedented manner (for example, by rationing commodities such as food, clothing and so on). The Emergency Medical Service, which took control of all health services for the duration of the war, showed that existing services were struggling and were of variable quality. It also demonstrated that it was feasible to organize health services nationally and collectively. By the end of the war it was generally accepted that the state should have a major role in the provision of welfare. The postwar reconstruction was built around the development of a welfare state, which was meant to be horizontally rather than vertically redistributive of wealth. That is, services funded through general taxation were not designed primarily to redistribute wealth from rich to poor, but to distribute costs and benefits over an individual's lifetime. Individuals would pay income tax while in employment in order to receive help during periods of unemployment or sickness.

The goal of postwar economic policy was full employment; unemployment was seen as a temporary phenomenon.

THE NATIONAL HEALTH SERVICE

The National Health Service (NHS) Act (1946) did not define 'health', 'illness' and 'care', and the responsibility of the state in regard to each. Comprehensive health care, free at the point of delivery, was promised but as Salter (1993, p. 172) points out: 'The political origins of these values reside in a model of health care which emphasised the obligation of public authorities to make provision for the community at large, rather than in a model centred on individual rights to health care'.

No curbs were put on the demands that could be made on the NHS. This led to a general public assumption that all needs could and should be met. There was also an implicit assumption that need was synonymous with want. These assumptions remained largely unchallenged until the 1970s.

The form that the NHS took in 1948 was largely the result of negotiation with the most politically powerful group in health care, the hospital consultants. Aneurin Bevan negotiated on behalf of the government. Hospital consultants were given a key role in policy making that was enjoyed by no other occupational group. Nurses were not involved in the negotiations, as it was largely assumed that they would accept the results, and would have no alternative but to join the new service. Nurses were seen as an occupational group that supported, and were subservient to doctors, and as such would automatically follow if doctors were persuaded into the NHS. Not surprisingly, given the marginalization of general practice, the NHS was structured as a sickness rather than a health service, and was dominated by the acute hospital sector.

Successive governments continued to increase spending on the NHS as the economy expanded in the 1950s and 1960s. Indeed, during both Labour and Conservative administrations between 1964 and 1974 social expenditure increased faster than economic growth. This was a time of consensus between the political parties in relation to state provision of welfare.

CHANGES IN THE 1970s

The end of consensus

Although there have always been critics of state welfare, in the postwar era their voices were somewhat muted. By the 1970s, however, both the political left and right felt that state welfare had not fulfilled its aims. The right considered that the 'Nanny State' had created dependency and stifled individual initiative. The left, on the other hand, argued that the state had not gone far enough in redistributing wealth. The impetus for the end of consensus, and the growing criticism of state welfare, was the oil crisis of 1973. Arab oil-producing countries quadrupled the price of crude oil, in protest against what was perceived as Western governments' support for Israel. Investment fell and the world was plunged into a major recession. Britain's weak economic position at the time, caused by 'stagflation' (a combination of stagnation and rapid inflation), meant that it was particularly affected. The postwar goal of full employment was no longer attainable. For the first time since the Second World War the inevitability and appropriateness of state provision of welfare was challenged.

Disillusionment with the inability of existing economic theory to provide a prosperous economy in the long term was accompanied by disillusionment with the institutions that had been spawned in its wake. This disillusionment led to the rise of the 'New Right' in British politics, and challenges to the dominance of medicine.

The rise of the New Right

The term 'New Right' was coined to distinguish the views of its advocates from 'old right' or traditional Conservatives (see also Ch. 2). Conservative ideology, as its name suggests, had been associated with the maintenance of tradition in the running of the country. New Right ideologists, on the other hand, in a revival of classic liberalism, sought to reduce the state's involvement in all areas of economic and social life. The New Right contended that Britain was in a state of government overload. They argued that the failure of both the economy and the welfare state was the result of increasing government intervention, which had led to inefficiency. The New Right placed great importance on the role of the family, which was seen as the natural provider of welfare services for its members, either by direct provision or by purchase on the open market. The New Right saw the solution to the failure of the welfare state through a return to the liberal ideas of the 19th century. They advocated placing a greater emphasis on the market, and a move from an interventionist to a minimalist role for the state. The New Right maintained that the state should be concerned only in those things, such as defence and law and order, which facilitate the smooth running of the market. A free market (i.e. free of government intervention) was perceived to be inherently superior because competition was thought to generate efficiency and maximize profit. The proponents of New Right ideology saw state-run agencies as being problematic because there were no in-built incentives to be efficient. There was no competition and no profit to be made. By the end of the 1970s the state institutions of welfare, which include the NHS, appeared to function more in the interests of their employees than in the interests of the service users. This had resulted in 'provider driven' services, where policy makers and professional groups decided which services would be produced, with little account taken of the wishes of consumers.

The goal of New Right economic policy is the reduction of inflation. This is achieved by reducing public spending, which allows a reduction in taxation. People can then keep more of what they earn, and make choices about the welfare services they wish to purchase. Within New Right ideology health care becomes a commodity to be purchased like any other. Inflation is kept low by low government spending, but the price is high unemployment, a price that is thought to be worth paying in order to stimulate enterprise and growth.

Private insurance schemes to finance health care needs have been advocated by many right-wing think tanks over the years, and the NHS review (Department of Health and Social Security 1989b) seriously considered this option. As yet, however, there has been no serious attempt made to alter the current means of financing the NHS. There is, on the other hand, according to Mishra (1990), considerable evidence that the Conservative government held down expenditure on the NHS in order to stimulate the growth of private health care.

The rhetoric of the New Right has proved, by and large, not to be borne out by events. Although low-income groups have suffered from cuts in the programmes and benefits,

universal services such as health care have been less vulner-
able.

FROM EQUITY TO EFFICIENCY

Equity, as a political concept, is broadly concerned with
fairness. In practice the use of the concept of equity in relation to health is usually taken to mean fairness in the *provision* of health care, rather than fairness in health status.
Although the 1946 NHS Act did not explicitly acknowledge equity as a key principle, it was an implicit aim
(Powell 1996).

Health policy in the 1970s was characterized by an attempt
to move resources from richer to poorer regions via the
Resource Allocation Working Party formula, and from well
funded to poorly funded client groups in the interests of
equity. The 1980s saw a change in direction from equity to
efficiency, which was more in line with New Right thinking.
Efficiency can be considered, broadly, as getting the best
value from available resources. Equity is sometimes hard to
reconcile with efficiency.

The new Conservative government of 1979 considered that
private sector skills and strategies should be transferred to
the public sector to improve efficiency. The assumption was
that NHS funding was adequate to meet the desired health
outcomes, but that resources were not being utilized
efficiently. The Conservative government believed that
introducing competition between providers, and incentives
and sanctions for employees would alleviate the problems
of stagnation and waste. Initially changes were made at the
periphery of health care delivery. These changes included
compulsory competitive tendering of those tasks that were

most open to casualization, such as cleaning, catering and laundry services.

The Griffiths management inquiry

Following changes in the management structure of nursing recommended in the Salmon Committee report in 1968 and the 1974 NHS reorganization, the authority and influence of senior nurses increased. The Salmon structure, as it was called, gave nurses a role in decision making at all levels and reduced the doctor's role in nursing matters. Nurses were represented at all levels of the consensus management structure.

The Griffiths management inquiry was set up in 1983 to consider ways of strengthening the management function within the NHS in order to improve accountability and value for money. It recommended that general management rather than profession- or occupation-specific management should be introduced. General management was designed to make doctors more accountable for their decisions but resulted in nurses losing their automatic representation at senior levels. As Walby et al (1994, p. 11) argue, 'the introduction of general management in 1985 reduced the status of senior nursing staff, and destroyed a career structure that had been exclusively available to nurses'. Davies (1995) comments that Griffiths ignored nurses because he did not regard them as important in decision making. Nurses were eligible to apply for general manager posts following their introduction, but as Levitt & Wall (1995) point out, few did, and even fewer were appointed. Davies (1995, p. 165) comments: 'Underlying the lack of developed expertise and the defensiveness and uncertainty of nurse managers themselves is surely a *failure to acknowledge that there is a management job to be done*' (original emphasis). Strong & Robinson (1990) argued that nurses were not educationally equipped to compete with administrators and doctors for senior management posts. Also, because nurses tended to take an equity or humanitarian stance over resourcing issues they were perceived to reject the managerial ethos of efficiency.

The NHS and Community Care Act 1990

By the late 1980s, despite the introduction of general management, doctors were still not perceived to be sufficiently financially accountable and so further controls were introduced under the NHS and Community Care Act 1990. For example, in order to increase financial accountability for clinical decisions, clinical directorates were introduced. In theory nurses were eligible for the post of clinical director, but in practice the vast majority of clinical directors appointed were medical consultants. The clinical directorate team, however, included a nurse manager and a business manager (since combined into one post in many instances), so nurses could influence planning and decision making, at least at the clinical level. But the wider agenda for health care and for nursing is still set elsewhere.

Managerialism did not stop the arguments about funding for the NHS. Matters came to a head in the autumn of 1987 with a number of highly publicized examples of cancelled operations and bed closures. In a BBC *Panorama* programme, the then prime minister, Margaret Thatcher, announced a wide-ranging review of the NHS, to report within 1 year. This was a clever tactic, albeit one that surprised her Cabinet, as it successfully bought time and, although the rationale given was that a review would be quicker than a Royal Commission, it also bypassed much of the normal consultation process. Evidence was not taken from professional or user groups, but from right-wing think tanks, monetarist economists (notably Alan Enthoven), and others who were likely to advocate a move away from state towards private provision. In the event, the review fought shy of recommending outright privatization. Instead the White Paper, *Working for patients* (Department of Health and Social Security 1989b), advocated the establishment of a market system within the NHS, which would separate the purchasing and providing roles in health care delivery. Similar market-style proposals were recommended for community care in the White Paper *Caring for people* (Department of Health and Social Security 1989a). Both White Papers were incorporated into the 1990 NHS and Community Care Act.

The internal market

The so-called internal market introduced under the NHS and Community Care Act 1990 was based on economic theories of supply and demand, in which knowledgeable consumers use their disposable income to purchase goods and services at a price which gives the best value for money. Producers of goods and services compete to give consumers what they want at a price that maximizes profit. The outcome of the perfect market is efficiency. The NHS, however, is not like a conventional market because there is no profit motive, and patients and clients do not directly purchase their own health care. General practitioners and health authorities act on their behalf. Because of this the NHS internal market is often called a quasi ('as if') market.

NHS trusts and the implications for nursing

Provider units, as suppliers of health care came to be known, were encouraged to apply to become self-governing trusts within the NHS. The first trusts, which were mainly in the acute sector, began operating on 1 April 1991. The last provider units gained trust status, or were merged, on 1 April 1996. GP practices with more than 11 000 patients (later reduced to 7000) were encouraged to become fund-holding and purchase care directly for their patients. NHS trusts were also given the power to set their own pay and conditions of working. In the early years these changes mainly concerned skill mix. The year 1995 did, however, see some attempts to link pay with changes in conditions of service (Cassidy 1995a and b). In the endeavour to remain competitive, and to attract contracts, trust managers began to look at the roles people carried out, and to consider whether they were appropriate, or could be done by someone less qualified. The results were quite diverse, ranging from very little change to a great alteration in the ratio of qualified to unqualified staff. Overall, though, the expected move towards the delivery of care by unqualified health care assistants, supervised by professionally qualified nurses has not materialized so far, but it is still very much on the agenda as NHS trusts seek to get value for money from expensive registered nurses. There were, however, many reported instances (albeit mainly anecdotal) of trusts attempting to save money by offering short-term or zero hours contracts to nurses (whereby the number of hours worked at any one time would be decided by the employer), and by the greater use of agency staff. Such strategies are designed to avoid the additional costs of employing people permanently. The fact that it would appear that short-term contracts are being used less frequently would suggest that, as nurses themselves warned, they are counterproductive. The fragmentation of nursing work, coupled with a lack of knowledge of, and commitment to, the employing organization by temporary staff can lead to less efficient care being given, and a poorer experience for patients (Walby at al 1994). This casualization of the workforce was not attempted with doctors, perhaps demonstrating that, as Davies (1995) and others have asserted, nursing work is undervalued and nurses are relatively powerless.

The use of agency nurses does not seem to have diminished and in some areas is increasing, which is of concern to many commentators. However, in many instances this is probably due to recruitment difficulties rather than being deliberate employment strategy. Castledine (1997) comments that team nursing, primary nursing and case management emphasize the importance of continuity of care, and yet the increasing number of agency staff is associated with a more functional or task-based approach to nursing care. Also, agency nurses may be expected to work in clinical areas where they do not possess appropriate skills or expertise (Castledine 1997; Snell 1997a). Interestingly, although there have been studies comparing the quality of care offered by qualified nurses compared with that of unregistered staff, little research has been conducted into the effect on patient care of the use of more temporary staff (Snell 1997b).

In some NHS trusts new posts and pay increases are dependent on accepting trust contracts, which are often less beneficial to nurses than the nationally agreed terms and conditions. An Income Data Services report (cited in *Health Service Journal*, news item, 28 Nov 1996, p. 7) stated that out of 87 NHS trusts surveyed, 42 gave staff less holiday and sick leave entitlement was generally reduced. In addition, a survey carried out for the Royal College of Nursing found that nurse executive directors on NHS trust boards were, on average, paid £6000 per annum less than their board peers, and half of those surveyed said that they were the lowest paid board member (Crail 1997a).

Future developments

How nurses' pay and conditions will be determined in the future remains unclear. The secretary of state for health has announced that there will be national pay awards in 1998/99, and no 'hybrids' incorporating local awards (Crail 1997b). However, the NHS Confederation is reported in the same article to be seeking enabling agreements, allowing NHS trusts to negotiate local terms and conditions in response to local labour market conditions, and there is much speculation that national agreements will specifically exclude those on trust contracts (Healey 1997).

There are fears that NHS trusts may seek to maximize efficiency by employing fewer highly educated nurses to deal with policy and strategic planning, and more low paid National Vocational Qualification (NVQ) trained support workers to carry out the majority of nursing work. This scenario is common in some industries, where an élite core commands high pay and conditions of service, and the vast majority of peripheral workers receive low pay and poor conditions. It could be argued that an élite is already developing in nursing, with roles that are given titles like 'clinician's assistant' and 'nurse practitioner'. These nurses often take over tasks previously performed by doctors, such as physical assessment and preoperative clerking, or manage their own case loads of patients with specific disease conditions such diabetes, hypertension and so on. Status is derived from the association with medicine and medical work, and the work involved is often delegated and largely routine. Once again decisions about nursing roles are being taken by others, with nursing largely acquiescing in the decisions made. The power to define nursing and to decide what is appropriately included as nursing work remains outside the sphere of nursing itself.

Often nurses can be seen simultaneously to gain and lose from health care developments whether these developments are generated from within the profession or outside it. Walby et al (1994), for example, highlight the fact that the professionalizing strategy of diploma level education for nurses has created a gap in service provision, which has been filled by NVQ trained staff. This training has offered an opportunity for many people, most of whom are women, to gain qualifications in health care work that might not have been available otherwise. However, it may also have undermined the professionalization strategy of nursing by creating a pool of partly qualified workers who are doing traditional nursing work for substantially lower salaries.

In the community, too, changes proposed in the 1996 White Paper *Choice and opportunity: primary care – the future* (Department of Health 1996), which is concerned with the deregulation of general practice, will have an effect on the relationship between nurses and other occupational groups. Christine Hancock (1996), general secretary of the RCN, suggests that this may offer opportunities for nurses to become involved in providing a wider range of services, and to become equal partners in primary care. She envisages the development of a new breed of 'supernurses', who will contract with GPs on a sessional basis to provide totally nurse-led primary health care (Hancock 1997). Salter & Snee (1997) see the situation rather differently, and argue that both Labour and Conservative party statements make it clear that doctors, and especially GPs, are the group that matters. As evidence they cite the slow progress being made in the field of nurse prescribing, which is still only at the pilot stage 5 years after the introduction of the legislation. Their argument is very persuasive because doctors more than any other occupational group in health care are seen to hold the key to cost containment. The major part of the NHS budget is composed of salary and capital costs which are difficult to reduce, so the potential for cost saving is largely limited to clinical costs. Salter & Snee further argue that nurses should accept the reality of the situation, accept medical power, and accommodate rather than challenge it. Some individuals with skills which are in demand and who are educated to a high level may well improve their position with this approach, but nursing as a whole does not benefit if the majority are not involved in setting the agenda for change.

The Labour government's White Paper *The new NHS: modern, dependable* (DOH 1997) announces a 10-year programme to modernize the health service which at first glance would appear to have much to offer nurses and nursing. These proposals signal the end of GP fundholding and the dismantling of the internal market. GPs and community nurses will form 'primary care groups' serving approximately 100 000 patients. These groups will control most of the NHS budget and will be responsible for allocating money for hospital and community services in their areas. The development of primary care groups appears to give both GPs and community nurses a major role in allocating resources to the local population.

ALTERNATIVES TO MODERN MEDICINE

Thus far this chapter has concentrated on the delivery of mainstream health care and the attempts to control its supply, but there is also pressure to control demand, mainly by exhortations from the government for people to adapt their behaviour and lead more healthy lives. In other words, people are being encouraged to take more responsibility for their own health. This is consistent with the New Right ideology discussed earlier, and coincides with increasing public disillusionment with medicine. A growing number of people are seeking alternatives to mainstream health care by joining self-help groups and seeking empowerment through consumer movements. The reasons for this are not entirely clear, but there is a growing pessimism about what medicine can offer. For example, although there have been some spectacular medical successes, such as renal transplantation and improved survival rates for some childhood cancers, the mortality rates for many common diseases have barely altered, and the chronic, degenerative conditions often associated with ageing are becoming more prevalent as the population lives longer. Perversely, some of medicine's successes have added to this public disillusionment, as people saved by technological advances survive with disability or increasing ill health.

Coward (1993) argues that there is a growing awareness that life events such as birth, illness and death have been mismanaged in a society where status and profit predominate. Williams & Popay (1994) add that modern medicine is becoming so reductionist in character that it ignores what is important to the person. The general public has become increasingly willing to challenge medical authority and its paternalism (benign or otherwise). There has also been a breakdown of the automatic trust awarded in previous generations to 'experts' generally, and the medical profession in particular.

At the same time, alternative or complementary therapies, including over-the-counter sales of health foods and herbal remedies, have become increasingly popular. Sharma (1995) found that one of the reasons people gave for using alternative medicine was the perceived inability of conventional medicine to cope with the social and experiential aspects of illness. Saks (1994) states that the term 'alternative medicine' reflects the predominantly outsider status of the disciplines within the British health care system, rather than the content of the therapies. This is also apparent in the lack of official research funding; yet medicine demands scientific evidence in support of claims of efficacy.

Others distinguish between 'alternative' therapies that are given instead of orthodox medical treatment, and 'complementary' therapies that are used as an adjunct to it. Some commentators recommend replacing the word 'alternative' with 'complementary' to reflect the growing collaboration between orthodox and non-orthodox practitioners, but Saks (1994) feels that this reconceptualization is politically inspired. Although those practitioners who have most interest in being acknowledged by medical orthodoxy may willingly accept the term 'complementary', there are still many practitioners challenging biomedicine philosophically. Saks cites acupuncture as an example; acupuncture is based on the use of meridians which bear little systemic relationship to the central nervous system.

Nurses and complementary therapies

Nurses have tended to use those therapies that are reasonably quick to learn, and rely on touch, massage and communication with the patient, such as aromatherapy and reflexology. Wright (1995) argues that nurses are attempting to humanize the health care system with the use of these 'high touch' complementary therapy techniques. Doctors, on the other hand, tend to favour long established and well-known therapies, and mostly use procedures such as acupuncture or osteopathy. Nurses also use complementary therapy in the context of general nursing care, either to supplement conventional therapy, to negate the necessity for invasive procedures, or to reduce stress. For example the use of massage and relaxation techniques may avoid the need for catheterization for urinary retention. Sharma (1992) states that nursing interest in some forms of complementary medicine may emanate from a desire to highlight the distinction between medicine and nursing.

Smith (1996) states that complementary therapies (by which he means those defined above as complementary and alternative) are being commissioned or provided by 60% of health authorities and 45% of general practitioners, particularly those that are fundholding. About £1 million is spent on them annually by the NHS.

EMPOWERMENT

A strategy that is increasingly being adopted by the public to counter the dominance of medicine on aspects of life such as pregnancy and childbirth and to encourage independence is consumer or user empowerment. The notion of empowerment is most developed in the field of learning disability, but other nursing disciplines are now attempting to catch up. Empowerment is concerned with enabling people to take control of their own lives, and the processes that enable them to do so. Baistow (1995, p. 34), has noted a 'lack of analysis of the meanings and practices that are associated with empowerment'. It is assumed that individuals or communities prefer to have control, and not devolve responsibility to professionals, and also that those in empowering roles do not have an *a priori* agenda. But as Grace (1991, p. 331) argues:

> *Although the [empowerment] discourse attempts to position the community as being 'in control', being the initiator, there*

is still an external agent in a background role that has controlling implications. The use of concepts such as 'enabling' and 'empowering' serves as a way of disguising this role. It appears as though the professional is facilitating what already exists in the community. On closer inspection it is possible to see the existence of a priori concepts of the professional that are directive and strongly implicated in the succeeding action.

This is because the planning is based on preconceived notions of how things should be, using the disparity in power and knowledge between professional and consumer or community groups. Baistow (1995) argues that in common usage the verb 'to empower' has lost its reflexive meaning. In other words empowerment is something done to you by a professional, rather than something you strive for yourself. It is not altogether apparent from literature on the subject just how empowerment will make a difference to the lives of those empowered. As Nettleton (1996) states, it is not clear what people are being empowered to do – make healthy choices? Demand political change? It is rather taken for granted that taking control of one's life is as much a priority for those being empowered as for those doing the empowering, and that being empowered provides the solution to problems that are in fact complex and multifactoral. As such it is becoming 'an ethical obligation of the new citizenry' (Baistow 1995, p. 37). Indeed, far from reducing the intervention of professionals into people's lives, Baistow believes that empowering people actually creates a niche for new forms of professional intervention such as facilitation. In other words empowerment is an agenda set by professionals, in which they decide who is an appropriate candidate for empowerment as well as the strategies to be employed in order to achieve it. Salvage (1992, p. 22) made a similar point regarding New Nursing when she argued that: 'The leaders of the New Nursing need to guard against the seductive assumption that empowering nurses is the route to empowering patients'. The converse is also true – empowering patients should not be used as a route to empowering nurses.

A recent nursing development which involves elements of empowerment is negotiated care planning. This involves developing treatment plans that are acceptable to the patient as well as the professional (Fradd 1997). While at the clinical level this may be possible, the impetus still comes from the professional, and it is still set within existing power relationships and the organizational structure of the NHS, where the patient is traditionally the least powerful player. The idea of empowering consumers by involving them in policy making has been addressed in unpublished research by Russell & Schofield (1994). They argue that incorporating consumer discourse into policy making in the absence of critical analysis may distort the phenomenon under discussion. The assumption made by researchers and policy makers is that people have realistic and adequate information about the alternatives available on which to make informed choices. However, in reality those who are using the consumer's view control the information received. These conclusions also apply to negotiated care planning. Who controls the information on which treatment decisions are made? Nurses need to be wary of the seductiveness of concepts such as empowerment unless they are really prepared to relinquish power themselves, and accept that the aims of the patient may not be those of the nurse.

RISK AND SURVEILLANCE OF THE 'NORMAL'

The 20th century has seen an increase in the observation of the healthy population through what Armstrong (1995,

p. 395) has termed 'surveillance medicine'. This trend has its roots in the 19th century visiting of the poor during epidemics, which set a precedent for inspection and surveillance that has now become accepted practice. Surveillance medicine dispenses with discrete categories of 'health' and 'illness' because it is concerned with the whole population. Health promotion capitalizes on the notion that health and illness are not mutually exclusive concepts. The healthy can become healthier and those with long term illness or disability often perceive themselves to be basically healthy. Armstrong (1995, p. 400), however, argues that 'such a trajectory towards the healthy state can only be achieved if the whole population comes within the purview of surveillance'. Surveillance medicine is closely related to the concept of risk. Although not new, risk has been redefined to mean an assessment of the likelihood of negative outcomes or adverse effects (Gabe 1995) or danger (Nettleton 1996). Risk increasingly refers to events outside the body, unlike signs and symptoms of disease, and is presented in the catchall of lifestyle: smoking is identified with heart disease and cancer, low fibre diets with bowel disease. Throughout history the major threats to health have come from factors outside of our control, but beliefs about the locus of control are now shifting to factors well inside our control (Skolbekken 1995). The focus of surveillance medicine is the 'pre-illness at-risk state. The risk factor, however, has no fixed or necessary relationship with future illness, it simply opens up a space of possibility' (Armstrong 1995, p. 401). With increasing constraints on budgets, health visitors in particular are being urged to abandon their universal approach to communities, and to target those populations deemed to be at risk. As more becomes known about the aetiology of disease and risk factors, nurses, especially when involved in health promotion, need to be wary of victim blaming and/or deterministic approaches where the possession of a risk is seen as leading inevitably to the disease itself. The ability to predict this with any degree of accuracy is, in most cases, poor.

The identification, and control or elimination of risk factors has attained considerable importance and prestige within health professions. Once risk factors become linked to causal factors, whether scientifically verified or not, they become subject to treatment, expanding the area of medical concern, as can be seen by the ever increasing number of articles on the subject in medical journals (Skolbekken 1995).

Risk and public perception

The general population has also adopted the idea of risk in relation to health, but here the idea of risk is more concerned with elements outside of our control. Some commentators (Waterfield 1996, Fitzpatrick 1996) argue that the public's obsession with risks such as bovine spongiform encephalopathy (BSE) and its possible transmission to humans, or with nut allergy or road rage, result from an overestimation of the scale of such problems and panic fuelled by the media.

Environmental concerns

Brown (1995), however, argues that the observations of populations living in areas of toxic hazard often precede official and scientific awareness, and these observations can trigger community action. On a small scale these have been concerned with issues such as road safety near schools, the dangers of dog excrement or discarded needles and syringes in public parks, et cetera. More prominent campaigns have included protests against the dumping of nuclear waste, and the existence of leukaemia clusters near nuclear power plants or electricity pylons. Lay involvement can identify cases of 'bad science' (Brown 1995, p. 101) and expose the limitations of science, leading to a general distrust of official science and a search for alternative sources of information. This has been a feature of the outbreak of BSE, and the subsequent, but not necessarily consequent, rise in the incidence of Creutzfeldt–Jakob disease (CJD) in humans, where the general public has largely mistrusted government and veterinary statistics and predictions. The official response to public alarm is often to criticize lay knowledge as unscientific, and to assume that scientific illiteracy on the part of the public is responsible for the anxiety (Grinyer 1995). In 1988, for example, aluminium sulphate solution contaminated the water supply of Camelford, a north Cornwall community. The committee of inquiry set up to examine the health consequences of the poisoning raised questions about the representativeness of those reporting continued health problems, and the evidence produced by the local community (cited in Williams & Popay 1994).

Brown (1995) describes toxic waste activists as different to activists in the environmental movement generally, as they usually enter via a personal experience, rather than from political commitment. As such they are typically working or lower middle class, and are motivated by the threat to their family's health, and lack of control over their environment. Williams et al (1995) describe a type of inverse care law, whereby those whose health is most at risk from environmental damage are those with least ability to mobilize resources to challenge the polluter. Membership of the environmental movement, on the other hand, has tended to be middle class. The environmental movement has tended to focus on global issues rather than local concerns. In the USA, the notion of environmental justice is a key concern and the toxic waste movement has been instrumental in highlighting the race, class and gender differential of the environmental burden. As yet, this issue has not really been addressed in the United Kingdom.

THE GLOBALIZATION OF HEALTH

We can no longer view specific ill health problems as being restricted to certain areas of the world. Events and hazards occurring far distant from the population concerned may affect health. The 1986 nuclear accident at Chernobyl, for example, affected crops and livestock in many countries outside the USSR. An awareness of such issues has increased the profile of the work of international health agencies. The most prominent of these is the World Health Organization (WHO), set up by the United Nations in 1948 to take responsibility for international health matters and public health. The WHO promotes health and a reduction in health inequalities through encouraging international co-operation and coordination of research (WHO 1992). The WHO formally acknowledged the link between health and the environment by setting up a Commission on Health and Environment (CHE) in 1990. The CHE expressed concern at the levels of premature death, particularly, but not exclusively, in less developed nations, caused by environmental agents such as contaminated water and chemical hazards in the workplace. Recommendations ranged from international agreements on the disposal of waste to local initiatives to ensure the provision of clean water, thus demonstrating the need to work both globally and locally.

The *World health report* (WHO 1997) identifies that the so-called 'diseases of civilization' have become more prevalent in developing countries as life expectancy increases and as lifestyles change to include the unhealthy behaviours of the industrialized world, like smoking. The report argues that disease needs to be fought on a global scale. Countries acting alone cannot tackle health issues such as, for example, AIDS. Increases in foreign travel facilitate the passage of disease from one area of the world to another. As travel becomes more rapid, the likelihood is that a person infected with a contagious disease in a foreign country will have returned home before symptoms appear. Indigenous populations may well have no resistance to many imported bacteria or viruses. Tourism can also cause health problems for the host country. For example, the high water usage in hotels will often deplete the supply available for the local area, and in areas prone to drought this can result in crop failure and famine.

Global warming

There are also global health problems, such as the need to reduce greenhouse gases, that no country has the power to tackle individually and which therefore require international action. The depletion of the ozone layer is a great potential health threat, yet no individual country can deal with it alone. It is not, however, just a matter of negotiating international agreements, because some nations are in a stronger position to effect change. For example, not all countries can afford to replace inefficient and polluting industrial processes with clean and efficient ones. If they were forcibly shut down this would affect the employment of millions of the world's poorest people and therefore their health. Similarly the destruction of the South American rain forest is being carried out largely to create cattle pasture to supply hamburger meat to the United States (Seitz 1995). For local people the need to secure an income is more important than preserving the environment. It also has to be remembered that because of high patterns of consumption, wealthy countries produce more of the gases that lead to global warming. People in developed countries use around 10 times more commercial energy than those in developing countries and burn over two-thirds of all fossil fuel, the largest source of greenhouse gases. It is only by tackling greenhouse emissions as a global issue, with those who are most polluting accepting the responsibility, and those who can afford to pay subsidizing the rest, that the problem can be addressed.

THE FUTURE

This chapter set out to explore the political issues concerning changing ideas about health and health care, and to examine their implications for nursing. Wright (1995, p. 15) has commented that 'predictions are inevitably fragile, based as they are on limited human vision for the unfolding possibilities'. Nevertheless, in view of the massive changes in conceptions of health and the provision of health care described here, I cannot conclude without some speculation as to the future of nursing and health care.

At the time of writing, the new Labour government has yet to operationalize many of its manifesto commitments for health. It has announced the end of the internal market in health care. The two-tier system produced by GP fundholding will be replaced by a fairer system of commissioning. However, the idea of competition between providers will not be abandoned (DOH 1997). Inequality is once again on the agenda, but the notion of efficiency has been preserved and both purchasers and providers are expected to effect value for money. There will not be a great increase in public spending. The private sector will continue to have the major role in the provision of long term care and will remain a significant employer of nurses. The private sector is also set to have a larger role in the financing of large capital projects for the NHS, such as building and equipping new hospitals. Although this is attractive in the short term as large NHS capital investments will not have to be met from public funds, the long term leasing costs which NHS trusts will have to pay to investors over many years may have an adverse effect on future clinical budgets.

Nurses have been promised that their numbers will increase as bureaucracy decreases, but the skill and grade mix of those extra nurses has not been made clear. Nurses need to be aware of the possible divisive effects of some highly educated nurses expanding their role into more medical tasks. This reinforces the notion that nursing can only gain status by its association with medicine, further devaluing the caring role, which for the majority of nurses continues to be central. There needs to be a distinction between those functions which nurses take on because they increase continuity of care and improve the patient experience, and those that are being delegated by the medical profession because they are considered mundane.

CONCLUSION

A new consensus appears to be emerging between political parties about the role of the state in welfare. Future nursing roles will need to encompass different conceptions of health and illness, and the blurring of the distinction between the two. As the general public have increasingly been encouraged to take responsibility for their own health this has led to a reappraisal of their relationship with professionals. Nurses, who are with patients 24 hours a day, and who are often the key workers in the community, are well placed to examine and renegotiate their relationships with the public. There is now, for the first time, a minister for public health, which may herald a move away from the dominance of curative medicine towards a collective attack on the causes of ill health. However, unless there is a radical reallocation of finances away from the acute sector and towards public health, and greater cooperation between the Department of Health and other government agencies, then a health, as opposed to sickness, oriented NHS will appear no nearer than it did in 1948.

■ QUESTIONS FOR DISCUSSION

- The changes which have taken place within the NHS over the past 18 years were designed to increase efficiency. To what extent have they succeeded?
- Will the state remain the major provider of welfare services in the future, or is it inevitable that the role of the private and voluntary sectors expand?
- Is the increasing specialization of nursing, with expanded and enhanced roles, a professional project that will add to the status of nursing, or a divisive tactic from which only a few can benefit?
- What are the costs and benefits of empowerment:
  - for clients and their families?
  - for nurses?

FURTHER READING

Midwinter E 1994 The development of social welfare in Britain. Open University Press, Buckingham

This book charts the development of social welfare from medieval times to the present, and focuses not only on health, but issues such as poverty, housing and education that have such a profound impact on health

status. It considers how the state has responded to social issues, and also the current questioning of the role of the state in welfare.

Paton C 1996 Health policy and management. Chapman and Hall, London

This gives a comprehensive account of the changes to the structure and management of the NHS, and also discusses alternative policy strategies. The issues considered include the internal market, purchasing, rationing and resource management. It will provide the reader with a clear understanding of current health policy debates.

Gabe J (ed) 1995 Medicine, health and risk. Sociological approaches. Blackwell, Oxford

The contributions in this book offer an appraisal of the personal and public health issues facing people in Britain and other industrialized nations. It considers the way in which people assess and manage personal and environmental risk, and the way in which formal organizations shape perceptions of, and manage, risk.

Davies C 1995 Gender and the professional predicament in nursing. Open University Press, Buckingham

Davies develops an illuminating analysis of the nature of nursing and the work that nurses do which is informed by feminist work on gender. The implications of current socio-political developments for the future of nursing are examined.

Trevelyan J, Booth B 1994 Complementary medicine for nurses, midwives and health visitors. Macmillan, Basingstoke

This is a practical book, which covers a range of complementary therapies including aromatherapy, Alexander technique, homeopathy and therapeutic touch. For each technique the use by, and implications for nurses is discussed, and there are also chapters which consider the growth of complementary medicine more generally.

REFERENCES

Armstrong D 1995 The rise of surveillance medicine. Sociology of Health and Illness 17(3):393–404

Baistow K 1995 Liberation and regulation? Some paradoxes of empowerment. Critical Social Policy 42(4):34–46

Brown P 1995 Popular epidemiology, toxic waste and social movements. In: Gabe J (ed) Health, medicine and risk. Sociological approaches. Blackwell, Oxford, ch 5, pp 91–112

Cassidy J 1995a Trusts act on pay deal. Nursing Times 91(9):5

Cassidy J 1995b NHS personnel chief sounds pay deal alert. Nursing Times 91(10):5

Castledine G 1997 Continuity of care vs the role of agency nurses. British Journal of Nursing 6(2):123

Coward R 1993 The myth of alternative health. In: Beattie A, Gott M, Jones L, Sydell M (eds) Health and wellbeing: a reader. Macmillan, Basingstoke, ch 10, pp 94–101

Crail M 1997a Nursing grudges. Health Service Journal 107(9 Jan):9

Crail M 1997b Playing the numbers game. Health Service Journal 107(29 May):13

Cronin J E 1991 The politics of state expansion. Routledge, London

Davies C 1995 The gender predicament in nursing. Open University Press, Buckingham

Department of Health 1996 Choice and opportunity: primary care – the future. HMSO, London

Department of Health 1997 The new NHS: modern, dependable. HMSO, London

Department of Health and Social Security 1989a Caring for people. HMSO, London

Department of Health and Social Security 1989b Working for patients. HMSO, London

Department of Health and Social Security 1990 NHS and Community Care Act. HMSO, London

Fitzpatrick M 1996 A mad, mad, mad, mad world. Living Marxism (February):14–15

Fradd E 1997 Negotiated care planning. Paper given as the 7th Professorial Nursing Lecture, University of Central England, Birmingham

Gabe J 1995 Health, medicine and risk: the need for a sociological approach. In: Gabe J (ed) Medicine, health and risk. Sociological approaches. Blackwell, Oxford, ch 1, pp 1–17

Grace V M 1991 The marketing of empowerment and the construction of the health consumer: a critique of health promotion. International Journal of Health Services 21(2):329–343

Grinyer A 1995 Risk, the real world and naive sociology. In: Gabe J (ed) Medicine, health and risk. Sociological approaches. Blackwell, Oxford, ch 2, pp 31–51

Hancock C 1996 What's in it for nurses? Health Service Journal 106(7 Nov):21

Hancock C 1997 Stand by for supernurse. Health Service Journal 107(9 Jan):17

Healey P 1997 A little local misunderstanding. Health Service Journal 107(21 Aug):12

Levitt R, Wall A (1995) The reorganised National Health Service, 5th edn. Chapman and Hall, London

Midwinter E 1994 The development of social welfare in Britain. Open University Press, Buckingham

Mishra R 1990 The welfare state in capitalist society. Harvester Wheatsheaf, London

Nettleton S 1996 Women and the new paradigm of health and medicine. Critical Social Policy 16(3):33–53

Powell M 1996 Granny's footsteps, fractures and the principles of the NHS. Critical Social Policy 16:27–44

Russell C, Schofield T 1994 Qualitative research in Australian health policy and service development: some pitfalls in emerging practice models. Paper given to the Qualitative Health Research Conference, Pennsylvania State University

Saks M 1994 The alternatives to medicine. In: Gabe J, Kelleher D, Williams G (eds) Challenging medicine. Routledge, London, ch 5, pp 84–103

Salter B 1993 The politics of purchasing in the national health service. Policy and Politics 21(3):171–184

Salter B, Snee N 1997 Power dressing. Health Service Journal 107(13 Feb):30–31

Salvage J 1992 The new nursing: empowering patients or empowering nurses? In: Robinson J, Gray A, Elkan R (eds) Policy issues in nursing. Open University Press, Milton Keynes, ch 1, pp 9–23

Seitz J L 1995 Global issues: an introduction. Blackwell, Cambridge, Mass.

Sharma U 1992 Complementary medicine today. Practitioners and patients. Routledge, London

Sharma U M 1995 Using alternative therapies: marginal medicine and central concerns. In: Davey B, Grey A, Seale C (eds) Health and disease: a reader, 2nd edn. Open University Press, Buckingham, ch 6, pp 33–44

Skolbekken J-A 1995 The risk epidemic in medical journals. Social Science and Medicine 40(3):291–305

Smith I 1996 More than pin money. Health Service Journal 106 (25 Jan):24–25

Snell J 1997a Temporary staff, permanent risk. Nursing Times 93(2):20–21

Snell J 1997b They're banking on you. Nursing Times 93(7):24–25

Strong P, Robinson J 1990 The NHS: under new management. Open University Press, Milton Keynes

Walby S, Greenwall J, Mackay L, Soothill K 1994 Medicine and nursing – professions in a changing health service. Sage, London

Waterfield B 1996 Beware nuts. Living Marxism (June):14–15

Williams G, Popay J 1994 Lay knowledge and the privilege of experience. In: Gabe J, Kelleher D, Williams G (eds) Challenging medicine. Routledge, London, ch 7, pp 118–139

Williams G, Popay J, Bissell P 1995 Public health risks in the material world: barriers to social health movements in health. In:

Gabe J (ed) Medicine, health and risk. Sociological approaches. Blackwell, Oxford, ch 6, pp 113–132

WHO 1992 Our planet, our health. Report of the WHO Commission on Health and Environment. World Health Organization, Geneva

WHO 1997 World health report, 1997. World Health Organization, Geneva

Wright S G 1995 Bringing the heart back into nursing. Complementary Therapies in Nursing and Midwifery 1:15–20

2

An introduction to political perspectives

Elizabeth Perkins

INTRODUCTION

The *Shorter Oxford English Dictionary* (OED) defines politics as: 'The science and art of government; the science dealing with the form, organisation and administration of a state or part of one, and with the regulation of its relations with other states' (OED 1987). Politics in post industrial society, and in particular in the second half of the 20th century, is as much about access to social power and personal empowerment as it is about government and political parties. Politics is increasingly about everyday life and in modern society most people are involved in some way in political processes. This involvement extends beyond support for political parties and voting in elections. As the feminist slogan 'the personal is the political' indicates, politics and political analysis also reach into the private spheres of relationships and the family.

Why should nurses be interested in politics?

In this chapter I will begin making the case for the relevance of politics and the political process to nurses and nursing. I will then explore the main political ideologies of liberalism, conservatism and socialism. It is the peculiar, but perhaps not unexpected situation that the positions of women, black people and minority ethnic groups, who historically have all suffered systematic inequalities, are rarely confronted head on in any of the major political theories. I will therefore also describe the sets of beliefs grouped under feminism and racism. Whether these beliefs qualify as cohesive ideologies is, however, disputed.

It is my aim, in each section of this chapter, to show how politics and political ideology have been translated into policies through which the institutions and practices relevant to health and health care delivery have emerged.

Definitions and ideologies

Before addressing the key political ideologies, it is important to define what we mean by ideology. Although subject to various interpretations, political ideologies are sets of ideas or beliefs that provide the basis for some kind of political action. Ideologies provide different ways of understanding the world, promote different solutions to economic and moral problems and shape the nature of political systems and governments.

The values and principles underlying political ideologies are often seen as ranged along a spectrum from left to right, in a linear procession from communism through socialism, liberalism and conservatism to fascism. This model oversimplifies the differences between each of the theories. In reality, these ideologies are not discrete and homogeneous categories; the values and ideas contained within them overlap, and the boundaries between them are blurred. Liberal ideas, for example, currently permeate both Conservative and socialist ideologies. To make matters more complex, within each ideology to be discussed in this chapter there are different traditions of thought. Liberalism can be divided into the strands of classical liberalism and modern liberalism; the former reflecting a belief in minimal state intervention in the lives of citizens and the latter reflecting the belief that the government should be responsible for the welfare of its citizens through the provision of a range of services such as housing, health and education.

It is important, therefore, to recognize from the outset that political ideologies are 'broad traditions of thought, which have evolved and developed under the pressure of changing historical circumstances and as a result of argument and debate and continue to do so' (Heywood 1992, p. 8). All political ideas are moulded by the social and historical context within which they emerge and as such are subject to moderation and change over time. For this reason, wherever possible, each political theory will be discussed within its relevant historical context.

THE CASE FOR POLITICS

Nurses, in as much as they are individuals, citizens, workers, consumers and predominantly women, are closely affected by the theory and practice of politics. Half of all women in employment are concentrated in three types of occupation: clerical and secretarial; personal and protective (which includes nurses); and sales (Sly et al 1997). The majority of nurses are employed within the National Health Service (currently about 356 000 nurses; DOH 1997) and nearly 90% of these nurses are women. The National Health Service is not only one of the largest employers in Great Britain but also a major consumer of public money. In 1996, 22% of government spending went on the NHS (Annual Abstract of Statistics 1996).

Despite the predominance of women in nursing, the positions women reach in the NHS do not reflect their numbers. In 1997 only 28% of chief executive or general manager posts were held by women (Labour Research 1997). When men attain higher and more senior positions than women in the same occupation this is known as occupational vertical segregation (Hakim 1979).

Politics not only affects the pay, conditions and employment of nurses, but is also central to the nature of the organization within which nurses nurse. Given the nature of nursing and the importance of nursing to health, nurses have much to contribute, both individually and collectively, to the direction of health and social care policies, to the development of their profession and to the environment in which they live.

Few policy decisions involving the NHS have occurred for abstract philosophical reasons. Major changes in the structure and delivery of health and social care services have served a number of different purposes, not always related to the promotion of health or the needs of service users. Changes in the provision of health and welfare occur when the external or the internal conditions, either alone or together, dictate it. For example, the NHS emerged in 1948 from a particular set of ideas and attitudes about the role of the state in the health and welfare of the population. The political and economic climate within which it has operated since its inception has transformed the nature of health care delivery while retaining some, but not all, of the principles which led to its development.

POLITICS AND THE NATIONAL HEALTH SERVICE

Although the present welfare state, and our expectations of it at the close of the 20th century, are very different from the model which grew out of the postwar settlement on welfare, the factors that have influenced these changes are crucial to understanding the role of politics in nursing and in health and social care delivery more generally.

Since its inception, the National Health Service has been through cycles of investment and cost constraint. As a major recipient of government expenditure, the NHS has had to compete with other government departments for funding. Competition has always been fiercest during periods of retrenchment in public spending. At the beginning of the 1950s, the Conservative government argued that the principles upon which it was founded should be re-examined on the grounds of cost. By the end of the 1950s a consensus on the importance of health and welfare provision had been reached by both Labour and Conservative ministers, result-ing in a tremendous growth in public expenditure (Digby 1989). By the 1960s it had once again become apparent that despite the expanding economy, expenditure on health was growing faster than the national income.

From the late 1960s onwards, welfare services, as the largest consumer of public funds, have come under continual scrutiny. As it became clear in the early 1970s that the post-war period of economic growth had ended, the politics of recession took over. For health care this has meant the more explicit rationing of services. As new budgetary restraints have been imposed by governments, attention has been diverted away from the previous aim of establish-ing a desirable level of health and social service provision for all.

Although there has always been some sort of consensus on the provision of welfare, the level at which it is fixed and the way in which it is administered have always produced divergences of opinion. The majority of changes that have been made to the structure of the NHS since 1948 have, however, resulted from political ideology largely shaped by fiscal crisis.

THE STATUS OF NURSING

Women historically have been the main healers in Western society: delivering babies, administering first aid and care on a paid and unpaid basis. Despite the importance of this, nurses have generally been accorded a relatively low status in society deriving from the links between women, care and concern for others. Within political theory, the role of women as carers is most frequently associated with a private dependent status which, while providing a foundation for our social structure, is commonly held to be part of women's oppression.

As Mary Wollstonecraft (1759–1797) and other early women's rights campaigners suggested, a concern for others involves self-sacrifice which ultimately militates against women's self-development and career prospects. Carol Gilligan (1982) suggests that while men profit from the care and concern of women, they promote the values of personal autonomy and individual achievement:

> *Women's place in man's life cycle has been that of nurturer, caretaker and helpmate, the weaver of those networks of relationships on which she in turn relies. But while women have thus taken care of men, men have in their theories of psychological development, as in their economic arrangements, tended to assume or devalue that care. When the focus on individuation and individual achievement extends into adulthood and maturity is equated with personal autonomy, concern with relationships appears as a weakness of women rather than a human strength. (Gilligan 1982, p. 17)*

Long hours and poor pay, in combination with the way in which care is devalued in our society, have traditionally maintained and promoted nursing as a vocation rather than as a professional career. More recently, however, with advancing technology and equal opportunities, there has been an attempt by nurses to achieve professional recognition for nursing.

The establishment of nursing as a profession depends upon a whole range of factors: breaking loose from the patronage of medicine and doctors, gaining a monopoly over the sphere of nursing practice and establishing the means to defend it (usually in law), and developing the means of educating, regulating and disciplining members are all essential components in this process. The emerging professionalization of nursing is demonstrated in a number of developments within nursing. These include the introduction of Project 2000, the growth of nurse specialist posts, nurse led prescribing and the development of a theoretical basis for nursing.

A number of critics identify problems with professional status as an occupational goal. Most notably, that professionalization usually discriminates against lower social classes and minority groups (Cross 1987, Davies 1995). Celia Davies's book, *Gender and the professional predicament in nursing* (1995), provides an excellent analysis of the predicament posed by the professionalization of nursing.

THE POLITICS OF COMMUNITY CARE AND FAMILY CARE

Nursing is not only the prerogative of trained NHS employees. This book could as easily have been entitled politics and care, to reflect the enormous contribution made to the care of sick, elderly and disabled people by family carers. The personal service that women provide in their caring role is often seen as an extension of their role in the family (Land & Rose 1985). As early as 1977, Patrick Jenkin, Conservative social services spokesman, claimed: 'The family must be the front line of defence when Gran needs help' (Jenkin 1977, cited in Coote & Campbell 1982, p. 85).

Family care, however, carries with it major implications for women, who bear the brunt of caring. Unlike trained nurses, family carers receive little, if any, appropriate financial remuneration for the specific quasi-professional tasks which they perform. Land & Rose (1985) attribute the lack of wage remuneration to the fact that family care is not distributed through a market nor administered by the welfare state. It has been calculated that unpaid carers provide a resource between £15 billion and £24 billion to the state (Kohner 1993). Informal carers remain part of the domestic economy, moulded by the relations which govern everyday life in the family and the community. Their presence is frequently used as the basis for limiting help and assistance from the statutory sector. By making a virtue of caring within the family, illness, disability and care all become private matters requiring private solutions:

> We know the immense sacrifices which people will make for the
> care of their own near and dear – for elderly relatives, disabled
> children and so on, and the immense part which voluntary
> effort even outside the confines of the family has played in
> these fields. Once you give people the idea that all this can be
> done by the state and that it is somehow second best, even
> degrading to leave it to private people (it is sometimes referred
> to as cold charity) then you will begin to deprive human beings
> of one of the essential ingredients of humanity – personal
> moral responsibility. (Thatcher 1978)

Community care has been a prominent policy goal since the Second World War and now, in the late 20th century, represents the linchpin of state welfare. While community care varies in practice according to the prevailing political ideology and economic climate, the philosophy behind community care has been tied to one particular view of community, a view of community which has been prevalent since the 1950s and 1960s.

Community occupies a sort of twilight zone, the common space which links the private world of home to the social world of living and working. For this reason it has been variously interpreted as geographical location, networks of relationships and networks of exchange. The concept of community indispensable to community care draws on all of these elements. It is of course geographic in the sense that it refers to the physical location outside of institutions. It is both the private world of home and the public space between home and institution. Inherent in this idea of community is a quality of human relationship which transcends the physical environment, bonding people together (Bender 1978) through family ties, identity, experience or interest.

It is this idea of community, enhanced by a reaction against the large institutions in which long-term care was carried out, which has proved so powerful an influence in the development of community care as a policy. In the abstract, the philosophy of community care appeared to be everything that institutional care was not: individual-orientated and humane. It claimed to deliver what sick and frail people wanted: a service provided in familiar surroundings by familiar people. It even appeared to be cheaper, although in fact it was never costed. From a service perspective, three different distinct types of care in the community have assumed prominence at different times: services provided in residential care; services provided through professionals working in the community; and services provided by the community on a voluntary basis (Allsop 1984, p. 108). However, in the 1990s, the reality is that 'community', as a prefix for care, represents little more than the care provided by the family and a way of reducing public expenditure, using the appealing rhetoric of community.

ETHNICITY AND NURSING

Just as women are a key feature of the NHS, so are people from different ethnic backgrounds. Recruitment of people from diverse ethnic backgrounds into nursing has been a feature of the NHS for the last three decades (Beishon et al 1995). From the early 1960s to the mid-1970s, the government sanctioned an overseas recruitment exercise to meet the chronic shortage of nursing staff in British hospitals. By 1971 there were 15 000 overseas nurses, of whom 40% were West Indian, 29% Asian and 27% African (Akinsanya 1988). At this time it was estimated that overseas nurses accounted for 9% of the hospital nursing population (Morton-Williams & Berthoud 1971).

Many of those entering nursing in the postwar period found themselves working as untrained nursing auxiliaries in the less popular areas of health care, notably in the care of elderly people and people with mental health problems and learning difficulties. Those who managed to gain a place on a training course were channelled into enrolled nurse courses as opposed to registered nurse courses. Once qualified, opportunities for promotion were restricted and appointment to senior posts frequently proved elusive. By the mid-1980s a combination of immigration restrictions and a declining need for non-indigenous labour brought the recruitment exercise to an end.

Concerns have more recently emerged in relation to the need for the NHS workforce to reflect the ethnic diversity of the local populations which it serves. Recent statistics show that the number of black nurses and midwives aged under 25 joining the NHS has fallen dramatically (*Independent*, 21 April 1997, p. 2). The reasons advanced for this decline in numbers are largely anecdotal and relate to discrimination at the point of entry, the influence of religious and cultural norms on career choice which may, for instance, direct Asian women away from nursing as a career, and the legacy created by the past, well-documented racist experiences of nurses and midwives from minority ethnic backgrounds working in the NHS. In the context of contemporary health and social care there is, however, an increasing need for the provision of services which meet the needs of a multi-ethnic society. The problems in recruiting and retaining nurses from diverse ethnic backgrounds have led to a reassessment of the way in which equal opportunity policies may be working in practice and have focused attention on the ways in which this trend may be reversed. Reversing the trend will inevitably take time and it is therefore imperative, many commentators suggest, given the importance attached by the nursing profession to the practice of holistic care, that all nurses develop an understanding of ethnicity which places specific ethnic identities within their own particular social, political, economic and material contexts (Baxter 1997, Gerrish et al 1995).

LIBERALISM

The roots of the Conservative philosophy which led to the substantial changes in the health service throughout the 1980s and early 1990s grew out of 19th-century liberalism. The late 20th century revival of interest in classical liberalism and in the idea of a free market economy is often referred to as neo-liberalism. It is the interpretation of liberalism by neo-liberal economists such as Milton Friedman (b. 1912) and Friedrich Hayek (1899–1992) that underpinned the reforms of the National Health Service by the

Conservative governments throughout the 1980s and 1990s.

Before Edmund Burke (1729–1797) there had been very little difference between liberalism and conservatism. As the influence of his political ideas spread across the European continent they met with the revolutionary movements of the 1830s and 1840s, polarizing opinion between those who supported the revolutionary ideals of liberty, equality, fraternity and those who opposed any form of social levelling.

The 'individual' is central to liberal theory. According to liberals such as Hayek (1967a), the natural state of 'man' (*sic*) is one in which he is free from regulation by the state and free to express his natural individualism. Any imposed order restricting personal liberty prevents the individual from attaining his or her potential (Hayek 1967b). 'Freedom preserves the opportunity for today's disadvantaged to become tomorrow's privileged' (Friedman & Friedman 1980, p. 89). All rules and regulations in society should, according to Hayek, exist solely to uphold and maintain an individual's freedom (Hayek 1967b). The total freedom of one person is automatically constrained by the equal, but different, freedoms of other individuals. Minimal social and political arrangements are therefore made to safeguard individual freedoms. It is an interesting paradox that acceptance of the imposition of these arrangements governing behaviour requires an identification on the part of the individual with the interests of others. Thus the individual is constrained from achieving total freedom by the recognition of the rights of other individuals. A current example of this would be the way in which smokers have their right to smoke in certain locations curtailed by the rights of non-smokers. The role which the government plays in establishing and implementing these arrangements varies both in theory and in practice. Friedman (1962, p. 27) states that the role of government is to arbitrate and enforce the agreed rules of society, while Hayek (1967b) believed that this was the function of the law and that the government should only act as an accessory to this process. Both agreed, however, that the paramount function of the government is to safeguard the natural rights of individuals to life, liberty and property and to minimize coercion. At different economic periods, liberal theory has been used or practised in different ways. Theoretically, in a period of economic expansion free markets become self-regulating and the generation of wealth is sufficient to develop and support a welfare infrastructure, either centrally administered or through private charities. Friedman & Friedman (1980, p. 171) cite the Rockefeller, Ford and Carnegie foundations as examples of philanthropic activity during a period of economic expansion in a free market economy. Tax deductible profits from these family empires were channelled into non-profit-making hospitals, privately endowed colleges and universities and many charities which aimed to aid the poor.

While liberalism appears to work well during periods of economic expansion, during times of recession the owners of production are put into intense competitive struggle for the acquisition of markets. Welfare and the material benefits conferred during an economic boom are cut or withdrawn. In order to maintain profit, wages are cut, as are standards of living. If the recession is accompanied by high unemployment, the threat to internal security of the country is increased and public order bills are passed to restrict the gathering and movement of groups of people in public places.

CONSERVATISM AND THE POLICIES OF THE NEW RIGHT

In Britain the nature of conservatism has changed enormously over time and has developed differently from that found in continental Europe. Conservatism can broadly be characterized by the defence of established customs and institutions, such as the monarchy, recognition of the importance of social order, authority, duties and obligations, the family and family values, and a hierarchical society in which different groups of people have different roles and responsibilities. The Conservatives who came to power in 1979 did not represent the traditional old-style paternalistic conservatism. They emerged from their years in opposition under the banner of the New Right with 'a militant hostility to ... the creeping collectivism of an overweening state' (Hall 1980, p. 4). The Britain that existed before the 1979 general election was characterized by nationalized industries, strong trade unions, a commitment to health and welfare expenditure and strong local government. In order for the New Right to achieve a free market economy, public spending had to be cut substantially and the state given powers to enforce government deregulation and privatization.

Under Margaret Thatcher and the political philosophies of the New Right, the postwar balance struck between the market-place and the provision of state welfare was overturned by an unbending commitment to the free market and to the restraint of public expenditure. In 1979 the language of the market-place entered the health and social care arena and choice, flexibility, competition, charging and contracts became key concepts in the management and running of the National Health Service. While law and order expenditure was increased, expenditure on health, housing and education was cut back; a matter of rolling back the state in order to strengthen it (Hall 1980).

The conservatism of the 1980s parts company with classical liberalism in its expression of social authoritarianism. That is, the authoritarian consensus on race, law and order and the family. Under classical liberal theory, the coercive powers granted to the government exist only for the purpose of achieving and maintaining a free economic system. However, the New Right used its power to introduce measures which threatened many democratic institutions. Alongside those policies which promoted unrestrained economic individualism, the government introduced new laws which restricted the definition of freedom and criminalized activities such as striking, demonstrating, picketing and in some circumstances even membership of a trade union.

Health and social care in the 1980s

Ideological opposition to social and public planning by the New Right placed the traditional practices of health and welfare in jeopardy. Health and social care were seen as commodities no different from any other commodity competing in the market-place. Innovation and experimentation believed to be optimal under conditions which favoured unbridled personal motivation, were said, by the New Right, to be stifled by the monopolistic hold the NHS had over the provision and practice of health and social care. Besides providing little incentive for advancing medicine, it was believed that the bureaucratic administration of the NHS fostered the conditions under which individuals could not readily be held to account, resources were wasted and personnel acted inefficiently and with relative impunity. In addition, because the state acted as an intermediary, employing a service on behalf of all prospective clients, the traditional relationship between producer and consumer was broken. Conservative governments of the 1980s viewed state-run services as restricting an individual's ability to make choices about the sort of services that he might require as well as constraining any comprehensive development of alternatives outside of that provided by the state. For as long as health and welfare services remained outside the market-place they were viewed by the right as having a destabilizing effect on the social and economic system, draining public expenditure and creating dependence in those who drew on them.

The liberal argument that 'nobody spends other people's money as carefully as they spend their own' was central to the criticisms of the NHS (Friedman and Friedman 1980, pp. 146–149). Services provided free at their point of consumption were deemed to encourage the consumer to over-consume. If people were made to pay for their services more directly, then only affordable services would be consumed.

Changes introduced in the 1980s

The 1980s were dominated by the debate about the level at which to fund health and social care, how it should be financed and how resources could be used more efficiently through changes to the delivery of services. Cost improvement programmes became a feature of all health authority accounting. Competitive tendering and the rationalization of patient services, which included the reduction in beds and patient facilities, contributed to substantial savings made throughout the health service. Swift and noticeable effects on service quality were recorded. A detailed report on the effect of the privatization of support services within NHS hospitals appeared in the *Guardian* newspaper: 'Each week we were issued with a definite supply of disinfectant, bleach, etc., which had been diluted to a minimal potency. If this ran out on the fifth or the sixth day, then the job had to be done with water only ... we were explicitly instructed by the management not to talk to the patients in the firm's time' (*Guardian*, 22 February 1984).

Management

One of the first most significant changes introduced by the Conservative government under Margaret Thatcher was the introduction of general managers. In 1982, Roy Griffiths, the deputy chairman and managing director of the supermarket chain, Sainsbury's, was brought in to give advice on the effective use of management and manpower in the NHS. The major recommendation was the appointment of general managers at all levels to provide leadership, introduce a continual search for cost improvement and change, motivate staff and develop a dynamic management approach.

Managers employed on short-term, renewable contracts quickly became the cutting edge of newly imposed budgets. The threat to managers of not having their contract of employment renewed was sufficient to ensure limited opposition to changes in the funding and delivery of services. Not surprisingly, the major concern of managers at this time was to keep within budget and balance the books (Harrison et al 1989). By the end of 1985 general managers were appointed at all levels of the service.

Purchasers and providers

In the White Paper, *Working for patients* (Department of Health 1989), the purchase of services was separated from that of the provision of services for the first time. By introducing an internal market, in which providers competed to sell their services to health authorities, it was hoped that services would become more responsive to patients and at the same time stimulate a greater efficiency in the use of resources.

MARXISM

The major stream of thought which came of age in the 20th century was Marxism. As will become clear, elements of Marxism underpin socialism. Karl Marx (1818–1883) was a German philosopher, economist and political thinker. His work provided the basis for much 19th-century socialist thought and greatly influenced communism in the 20th century. In fact, Hobsbawn identifies Marxism as the intellectual justification and inspiration of communism: 'The collapse of the USSR naturally drew attention primarily to the failure of Soviet Communism, that is to say, of the attempt to base an entire economy on universal state ownership of the means of production and all-encompassing central planning, without any effective recourse to market or pricing mechanisms.' (Hobsbawn 1995, p. 563).

Marx developed complex and systematic theories involving the laws of history and the development of civilization. According to Marx, class conflict was the key to understanding human history and society. As a consequence Marxism is constructed around the relations of appropriation and exploitation and the primary contradiction between labour and capital. Marx's analysis centres on the alienation of capitalist productive processes. Marx argued that capitalism and the industrial process had alienated human beings from their own skills and talents through their involvement in a productive process geared towards the creation of profit. Not only are workers distanced from the things they produce but capitalism demands that at work they are also distanced from the people with whom they work. Rewards are tailored to the individual and personal advancement relies on self-promotion and self-interest.

With the beginnings of commodity production, human labour assumed a monetary value in the market-place. The sale of labour took the worker out of the community and for the first time created a division between the world of business and industry and the world of the family. Whilst the productive process alienated the worker from work, it also brought about a spatial separation between the worker and his family. The woman, remaining in the home, became a non-producer. This split between the public and private worlds of work and home provided the material conditions for the subsequent devaluation of women. Traditionally, Marxist analysis has centred on men and their relationship to the means of production, or, more specifically, on men as commodity producers and as wage earners. Women only figure in this analysis in as much as they have the theoretical potential to be labourers or producers. It is only more recently that post-Marxian theorists such as Gramsci have begun to tackle the vast complexities of oppression, domination and subservience and their reproduction through parenting, education, culture and socialization (Vogel 1983).

According to Marxist philosophy, with the emergence of capitalism the family began to function as a repressive institution of the state, helping to maintain the perpetuation of the unequal distribution of wealth and the ownership of productive resources. Doyal & Pennell (1983) identify a number of ways in which the capitalist system creates contradictions between health and profit. Although in the developed world capitalism has provided the basis from which the average life expectancy has increased, it has also produced the conditions for the development of new health problems. The effects of shiftwork, overtime, and the use of toxic chemicals and materials on the workforce are well documented. Doyal also points out that not all people are affected equally by these processes, as evidenced by the class differences in morbidity and mortality. 'Working-class people die sooner, and generally suffer more ill health than do middle-class people' (Doyal & Pennell 1983, p. 26).

Marxist theories quite tightly document a historical analysis of the woman's changing role which feminists, most frequently, but not exclusively, have built on in an attempt to develop a political analysis of the role of women. Just as the family is central to class-based society, so, feminists argue, is the oppression of women crucial to the family. In order to keep the wife at home, women are excluded from a central productive role. They become economically dependent on men or on a man, and they are discriminated against in educational and job opportunities and conditioned into an acceptance of this as their lot. However, within Marxism, women's struggles are subordinated to class struggles in such a way that the oppression of women cannot be resolved without major changes in the nature of the capitalist economy.

For Engels, as for succeeding generations of Marxists, the oppression of women is structural, having simply an economic cause and an economic solution. For this reason, Marxism does hold out the possibility for the role of women to change; should capitalism demand a labour market made up of low-paid female workers and unemployed deskilled men, a Marxist analysis would envisage women assuming such an economic role. Whether or not men would become primary carers given the 'right economic circumstances' (whatever they might be) is, however, questionable. De Beauvoir cautions against placing hope in a purely economic revolution as women's salvation.

> *We must not believe ... that a change in woman's economic condition alone is enough to transform her, though this factor has been and remains the basic factor in her evolution; but until it has brought about the moral, social, cultural and other consequences that it promises and requires, the new woman cannot appear. ... This she could only do through a social revolution. (De Beauvoir 1949, p. 734)*

SOCIALISM

Socialism is perhaps one of the broadest ideologies. It embraces a number of different political theories resulting in different interpretations of the goals of socialism and of the ways in which those goals are best achieved. The roots of socialism lie in the 18th and 19th centuries, when it developed as a reaction to the social and economic conditions generated by the growth of industrial capitalism. In particular, early socialism was influenced by the harsh and often inhuman conditions in which the industrial working class lived and worked. Socialism was seen by communists and others as a transitional strategy towards an equal and utopian society.

Socialism in Britain

The Fabian Society, formed in 1884 and led by Sidney and Beatrice Webb, had a greater impact on British socialism than did Marx. The Webbs were important social reformers who advanced the idea that socialism was to be achieved through political action and education. The founding of the British Labour Party in 1918 was designed to fulfil these functions.

The basic principles to which socialists ascribe identify the individual as inseparable from the rest of society. Cooperation rather than competition characterizes the natural relationship between individuals with the incentive to work hard deriving from the desire to contribute to the common good. Socialism is founded on the belief that although people are not born equal, most human inequality results from different experiences in society. Human nature can be moulded by social circumstances; social equality can therefore be achieved by redistributing wealth to enable people to develop their full potential. While Conservatives would argue that individuals are essentially self-seeking, socialists would argue that society encourages and rewards selfish behaviour.

Traditionally, socialists have linked their views to the interests of the working class. Class is used to denote a group of people sharing a common economic position. On the basis of this it is assumed that people of the same class experience similar working and social experiences. In 1881 class was an important criterion for admission to the Nightingale Fund Training School. The class criterion guaranteed that prospective nurses did not 'come from the same ranks as the rough domestic servants or the paupers upon whom the nursing in the workhouse had been based' (Davies 1980, p. 88). This continued in nursing until the 1970s.

The working class is the class of people to whom socialists have traditionally looked in order to achieve social change and even social revolution. As modern methods of production and technology have advanced, it is by no means clear that the working classes as previously defined still exist in the same way or constitute the backbone of support for the Labour Party today.

New Labour

Thatcher proclaimed the death of socialism when the Labour Party was defeated in 1983. In reality, since the 1950s there has been a gradual movement in socialism towards social democracy and an acceptance of capitalism. The concept of social democracy originally referred to the collective ownership of productive wealth and the achievement of a classless society. More recently it is used to reflect a balance between the market economy and state intervention in which capitalism is modified to take into account the principle of social justice.

Rising from the ashes, New Labour signals a further development in the ideology of socialism on which it is based. Under the leadership of Tony Blair, socialism has been adapted to accommodate market economics. In its 1990 document *Looking to the future* (Labour Party 1990), Labour acknowledged the central role played by the market economy in producing and distributing wealth. Gone is the emphasis on social ownership and Clause IV (the common ownership of the means of production, distribution and exchange). Instead the emphasis is on public–private partnerships and the efficacy of markets.

New Labour's policies on health and social care

One week after the election, on 9 May 1997, Frank Dobson, secretary of state for health, in his address to senior NHS executive staff, stated that the Labour Party was committed to ending the internal market in health care and the two-tier service which favoured patients attached to GP fundholding practices (Department of Health 97/091). It was generally considered that the internal market had failed to deliver the benefits usually attributed to markets, such as reduced costs, increased quality of care and responsiveness to patients' needs.

In confirming a wide ranging review of health service expenditure, Dobson announced that the review would consider a range of options including means-tested fees for visits to GPs and hotel charges for hospital care.

It was not until December 1997 that the Government launched its plans for the NHS. Entitled the *New NHS: modern, dependable* the White Paper outlined radical reforms for health care delivery. Central to the reforms is the integration of care outside the hospital. The majority of health care commissioning is to be delegated to locality groups of general practitioners and their primary health care teams. New primary care groups (PCGs) will serve populations of about 100 000 people through a unified cash-limited budget.

Primary care groups are not to be free standing unaccountable entities. PCGs will be directly accountable to Health Authorities (HAs), and will be expected to deliver and commission services within the framework of Health Improvement Programmes. Health Improvement Programmes are to be drawn up by HAs in consultation with PCGs, local populations and other local organizations and will address the targets outlined in the Government's Green Paper on public health entitled *Our Healthier Nation. A Contract for Health* (Department of Health, 1998).

Local authorities will be formally represented on PCG boards. Other PCG board members will include community or practice nurses, a lay member, a HA non-executive and a PCG Chief Office/Manager (HSC 1998/139).

Although the White Paper identified four levels at which a PCG might operate, depending on the amount of responsibility to be assumed for the commissioning and provision of community health services, it is envisaged that most PCGs will begin by supporting Health Authority commissioning of services (Level 1) or by taking devolved responsibility for managing the health care budget (Level 2).

Other crucial elements of the new reforms include the pursuit of effective clinical care through the creation of evidence-based National Service Frameworks which will bring together the best evidence of clinical and cost-effectiveness to ensure consistency of access to high quality care. A new National Institute for Clinical Excellence will draw together the evidence on clinical and cost-effectiveness and will ensure the dissemination of information and guidelines to all parts of the NHS. Locally, the existing systems of professional self-regulation are to be strengthened through the introduction of clinical governance.

The White Paper was strong on rhetoric but less clear on exactly how PCGs would operate. Since the launch of the

White Paper much energy has been invested in discussions around the nature and configuration of PCGs in order to meet the July 1998 deadline for agreeing boundaries. By 6 August 1998, 480 PCGs had been agreed covering populations ranging from 50 000 to 220 000. The groups will operate in shadow form until April 1999 when GP fund-holding will be brought to an end (Department of Health, 98/327).

FEMINIST THEORIES

The term 'feminism' is thought to have first come into use as late as the end of the 19th century (Offen 1985). However, demands that women be accepted as rational human beings capable of self-determination and of living with equal civil and political rights predate the coining of this term. In Britain, Mary Wollstonecraft began the debate with the publication in 1792 of her treatise *A vindication of the rights of woman*. In it she challenged the idea that human rights and freedom applied only to men.

While the study of patriarchy and the family have largely been central to the feminist construction of women's oppression there is no single body of work that can be called feminist theory. The feminist movement itself is racked with ideological debates about the analytic primacy and independence of male domination over class and race, over definitions of patriarchy and the role of production in the oppression of women. It is these differences that impede unity under the banner of gender among all feminists, let alone all women.

At its lowest common denominator, it could be said that underlying all feminist debate is the belief that gender is not simply the difference between the sexes but represents the division, oppression, inequality and the internalized inferiority of women on the basis of sex (Barrett 1985). However, feminist theory that looks for the status of trans-historical theory as a way of explaining this position of women almost inevitably relies on other theoretical frameworks which, on the whole, provide inadequate explanations of women's oppression.

Patriarchy

Patriarchy, the system of social structures and practices in which men dominate, oppress and exploit women (Walby 1990, p. 20), appears as a self-evident piece in the jigsaw puzzle of capitalism, neatly dovetailed by the functional fit of women into the family for this role. There is no theoretical space within Marxist philosophy to develop an understanding of patriarchy, either as a separate or a related system, because the woman question is almost inevitably collapsed into the question of class.

Firestone's (1972) critique signals the concerns held by a number of feminist writers about a purely materialist Marxist analysis of the position and role of women. She argues that there is a level of reality which does not stem directly from economics. 'The assumption that beneath economics, reality is psychosexual is often rejected by those who accept a materialist view of history because it seems to land us back where Marx began; groping through a fog of utopian hypotheses, philosophical systems that might be right, that might be wrong ... systems that explain concrete material developments by a priori categories of thought' (Firestone 1972, p. 15).

The very nature of theorizing is seen by some feminists as

an essentially male activity, the majority of philosophical and ethical theories from which women have been excluded being male conceptions. There is, therefore, a movement within feminism which resists any attempt at a theoretical understanding of the position of women and especially of adding themselves into current or prevalent theories. This, it is said, results in women adding themselves in on men's terms (Gross 1986, p. 193). Taken to its extreme, it is argued that language and meaning itself are male constructions and thereby 'de-scribe' women (Daly 1978).

Biology and reproduction

Some feminist theorists accept language as common and adapt (essentially male) political theories to explain more fully the position of women. Figes (1972) identifies capitalism as the root cause of the modern social and economic discrimination against women. At the crux of her analysis lies the issue of paternity and the need for the man to ensure paternity over his child(ren).

> *Once a man knows, that there is a physical link between himself and the child in his woman's womb, that provided no other man has been allowed to impregnate his woman, the child will definitely be his. ... Reliance upon the fact that the child is his can only be exacted by control of the woman since his sphere over other men is more problematic. (Figes 1972, p. 39)*

According to Figes's analysis this requires that men have both mental and physical control of women. The solution that Figes favours is the liberation of women from marriage which makes her an appendage to man, with the corollary that children should become the primary responsibility of the state.

Other feminists begin with patriarchy as the universal fundamental system of domination. Firestone (1972) attempts to develop a view of patriarchy grounded in the biological reproductive capacity of women. She argues that the sexual imbalance of power is biologically based and that men and women were not created as equal.

It is upon this 'natural' reproductive division that the class-based division of labour as well as the 'paradigm of caste' (discrimination based on biological differences) are based. Firestone promotes the family as the primary unit through which patriarchy and the male/female divisions emerge. Women's reproductive biology makes women dependent on men for survival through the dependence of children upon her for their survival.

Firestone does not believe that biology is immutably determining; it can be transcended by political action. This entails the recapturing of the means of reproduction through the repossession of women's bodies by women, the control of human fertility, and freedom from reproduction through intrauterine pregnancy.

In presenting the reproductive function as the impediment to emancipation, Firestone colludes with the male dominated ideology that devalues the skills of childbirth and child rearing and favours driving ambition, competition and emotional detachment. For women to gain equality they must become men. The flaw in Firestone's analysis is most apparent in its conclusion, that freeing women of their reproductive function through extrauterine pregnancy will destroy the basis of their inequality. Unless the balance of power is changed before women hand over responsibility for bearing children, the control of extrauterine pregnancies will most likely be assumed by men. An historical analysis of the development of midwifery highlights the way in which men have assumed a major role in the field of obstetrics and gynaecology (Ehrenreich & English 1974). Unless there is a mechanism whereby women remain in charge of reproduction without having the responsibility, or suffering the social consequences of rearing children, any advance in technology will almost certainly give greater control to men.

Feminism and nursing

Given the predominance of women in nursing it might be expected that nurses would form an easy alliance with feminism. However, as has been shown in this section, feminism embraces a number of different perspectives, few of which reflect the position of women who choose to care on a paid basis. While the practice of feminism often revolves around very practical issues, for instance the wages for housework campaign, many aspects of feminist theory are couched in abstract and inaccessible language and draw on an élite group for their appeal. In some feminist theories nursing itself is characterized as an embodiment of everything that feminism opposes; a female occupation in a male dominated culture; the nurse as the doctor's handmaiden. As more women enter the medical profession the position of women as nurses may be better understood within other theoretical frameworks.

RACISM

There is no unified ideological construct which has racism as its cornerstone. Although racism predates fascism, it is often discussed in the context of fascism. Fascism emerged during the 19th century but achieved its peak in Europe between the two world wars when it drew support predominantly from the lower middle classes. In contrast to liberalism, conservatism and socialism, fascism is not based on a well articulated theory, for instance it has no clear or well articulated views about the economy. As Heywood highlights, fascism is frequently better known for what it stands against than for what it positively supports. It is anti-rational, anti-liberal, anti-capitalist, anti-bourgeois and anti-communist (Heywood 1992).

Put at its most simple, racism is based on the following assumptions:

- humankind can be divided into different races on the basis of biological or genetic characteristics
- racial divisions are of political significance, more important than analyses based upon class, gender or nationality.

Nurses' experience of racism

Institutional racism is still manifest in many aspects of the National Health Service today. Maslin-Prothero (1994, p. 171) makes the distinction between 'direct discrimination', where someone is dealt with less favourably on racial grounds, and 'indirect discrimination', where policies and practices have a discriminatory effect even though it may be unintentional. Recent studies have identified both these types of discrimination within the NHS.

In a study of over 14 000 nurses carried out by Beishon et al (1995), researchers found that discrimination was thought to operate at all stages of the recruitment, training and promotion of nurses and midwives. Access to middle-ranking clinical posts (up to grade E) was less of a problem than access to the more senior posts (grade F and above). Beishon et al also found that there were far fewer minority ethnic nurses in midwifery and children's specialties than there were in mental health, elderly care and medical and surgical areas. In addition, a large proportion of black and minority ethnic nursing staff had experienced racial harassment from patients and, to a lesser extent, from nursing colleagues and management. Although this harassment constituted a regular feature of working life, few incidents were reported to senior management in the belief that little effort was being made to deal with the problems of racial harassment.

Patients' experience of racism

Just as important as the experience of nurses in the National Health Service is the experience of people of different ethnic origins as patients. There is increasing research evidence to suggest that ethnicity plays an important role in the health, diagnosis, treatment and care of minority ethnic groups.

A study of the health of Britain's ethnic minorities showed that ethnicity has an impact on the quality of health care received by patients with relatively low rates of referral of ethnic minority people to secondary health care (Nazroo 1997). While the author argues that much of the 'ethnic variation' in health results from differences in socioeconomic position (Nazroo 1997) the position is less clear when mental health is considered. African-Caribbean males and females appear to be more likely to be admitted to hospital with a psychiatric diagnosis and once admitted are more likely to be diagnosed as schizophrenic (Dean et al 1981) and to receive harsher forms of treatment than equivalent white groups (Cope 1989). These findings have raised doubts about whose interests are best served by the practice of psychiatry in society today (Frances et al 1989).

Interpreting the evidence on the utilization of health and social care services by minority ethnic groups is complex. Great variation in use has been recorded in relation to specific minority ethnic groups and in relation to different types of service. Utilization rates alone reveal little about demand or need for service, the frequency with which a service is received or the quality of the service received. Clearly, however, there are a number of factors which restrict access to services and which are more likely to affect particular minority ethnic groups. These include: a lack of knowledge of the range and extent of service provision; communication difficulties; culturally insensitive services; and the propensity of services to be rationed according to commonly held and often inaccurate assumptions which work against the receipt of services by particular ethnic groups – one such assumption being that extended Asian families prefer to look after their own family members (Gunaratnam 1993).

CONCLUSION

Welfare provision and policy in Britain have a history of being a flexible response to a particular set of economic and social circumstances. That is to say that although, over time, massive gains have been made in welfare policy, the relationship between 'need' and 'service provision', whether at the individual or population level, is a complex one. Which issues appear on the policy agenda, who stands to benefit and what they stand to gain have, in the past, had as much to do with issues of political ideology, social control and cost as with illness or destitution.

■ **QUESTIONS FOR DISCUSSION**

- What is the relevance of politics and political processes to nurses and nursing?
- Why are women still under-represented in senior nursing posts?
- Why is community care portrayed as care on the cheap?
- In what respect do the ideologies of liberalism, conservatism and socialism overlap?
- Are the policies of New Labour designed to attract the working class vote?

FURTHER READING

Ham C 1992 Health policy in Britain: the politics and organisation of the National Health Service, 3rd edn. Macmillan, London

This book provides an assessment of the current state of the NHS and the impact of politics on its structure and the nature of health care delivery.

Heywood A 1992 Political ideologies: an introduction. Macmillan, London

This book describes in detail the major Western ideologies. It provides clear and accessible descriptions of the historical development of these ideologies and provides an analysis of their use in contemporary society.

Skellington R, Morris P 1992 'Race' in Britain today. Sage, London

This book contains a wealth of information on the experiences and lives of minority ethnic groups in education, the labour market, health, welfare, housing, and the criminal justice system.

Davies C 1995 Gender and the professional predicament in nursing. Open University Press, Buckingham

This book examines the predicament for nursing of professionalization. It explores the consequences of professionalization for the laity in general and examines the potential impact of professionalization on nurses and nursing.

REFERENCES

Akinsanya J 1988 Ethnic minority nurses, midwives and health visitors: what role for them in the National Health Service? New Community 14:444–450

Allsop J 1984 Health policy and the National Health Service. Longman, London

Barrett M 1985 Women's oppression today: problems in Marxist feminist analysis. Verso, London

Baxter C 1997 Race equality in health care and education. Baillière Tindall, London

Beishon S, Virdee S, Hagell A 1995 Nursing in a multi-ethnic NHS. Policy Studies Institute, London

Bender T 1978 Community and social change in America. Rutgers University Press, New Brunswick, NJ

Coote A, Campbell B 1982 Sweet freedom. Pan Books, London

Cope R 1989 Compulsory detention of Afro-Caribbeans under the Mental Health Act. New Community 15(3):343–356

Cross E 1987 Observations on Project 2000. Radical Nurses Newsletter, Spring Issue, Sheffield, Yorkshire

Daly M 1978 Gyn/ecology: the metaethics of radical feminism. Beacon Press, Boston

Davies C (ed) 1980 Rewriting nursing history. Croom Helm, London

Davies C 1995 Gender and the professional predicament in nursing. Open University Press, Buckingham

Dean G, Walsh D, Downing H, Shelley P 1981 First admissions of native born and immigrants to psychiatric hospitals in south east England, 1976. British Journal of Psychiatry 139:506–512

De Beauvoir S 1949 The second sex. Penguin, Harmondsworth

Department of Health 1989 Working for patients. HMSO, London

Department of Health 1997 Health and personal social services statistics for England: 1996 edition. HMSO, London

Department of Health 97/091 Frank Dobson announces action to end the two tier National Health Service, Friday 9 May 1997

Department of Health 1997 The New NHS: modern, dependable. HMSO: London

Department of Health 1998 The new NHS: modern and dependable: developing Primary Care Groups. 13th August (HSC 1998/139)

Department of Health 1998 Minister welcomes formation of 480 Primary Care Groups. 6th August (HSC 98/327)

Department of Health 1998 Our healthier nation. A contract for health. HMSO: London

Digby A 1989 British welfare policy: workhouse to workfare. Faber and Faber, London

Doyal L, Pennell I 1983 The political economy of health. Pluto Press, London

Ehrenreich B, English D 1974 Witches, midwives, and nurses: a history of women healers. Glass Mountain Pamphlet No. 1, London

Figes E 1972 Patriarchal attitudes: women in society. Panther, London

Firestone S 1972 The dialectic of sex: the case for feminist revolution. Paladin, London

Frances E, David J, Johnson N, Sashidharan S 1989 Black people and psychiatry in the UK. Psychiatry Bulletin 13:482–485

Friedman M 1962 Capitalism and freedom. University of Chicago Press, Chicago

Friedman M, Friedman R 1980 Free to choose: a personal statement. Penguin, Harmondsworth

Gerrish K, Husband C, MacKenzie J 1996 Nursing for a multi-ethnic society. Open University Press, Buckingham

Gilligan C 1982 In a different voice: psychological theory and women's development. Harvard University Press, London

Gross E 1986 What is feminist theory? In: Pateman C, Gross E (eds) Feminist challenges: social and political theory. George Allen and Unwin, Hemel Hempstead, pp 190–204

Guardian 1984 (22 February 1984)

Gunaratnam Y 1993 Breaking the silence: Asian carers in Britain. In: Borrat J, Pereira D, Pilgrim J, Williams F (eds) Community care: a reader. Open University Press and Macmillan, London, pp 114–123

Hakim C 1979 Occupational segregation: a comparative study of the degree and pattern of the differentiation between men and women's work in Britain, the United States and other countries. Research Paper 9, Department of Employment, London

Hall S 1980 Drifting into a law and order society. Cobden Trust Human Rights Day Lecture, 10 December 1979

Harrison S, Hunter D, Marnoch G, Pollitt C 1989 The impact of general management in the NHS. University of Leeds and the Open University, Buckingham

Hayek F A von 1967a The economy, science and politics. In: Hayek F A (ed) Studies in philosophy, politics and economics. Routledge, London, pp 251–269

Hayek F A von 1967b Principles of a liberal social order. In: Hayek F A (eds) Studies in philosophy, politics and economics. Routledge, London, pp 160–177

Heywood A 1992 Political ideologies: an introduction. Macmillan, London

Hobsbawn E 1995 The age of extremes: the short twentieth century: 1914–1991. Abacus, London

Independent 1997 (21 April 1997), p 2

Kohner N 1993 A stronger voice: the achievements of the carers' movement 1963–1993. Carers' National Association, London

Labour Party 1990 Looking to the future. Labour Party, London

Labour Research 1997 Women knock on the boardroom door. 86(1):125–138

Land H, Rose H 1985 Compulsory altruism for some or an altruistic society for all? In: Bean P, Ferris J, Wynes D (eds) In defence of welfare. Tavistock, London

Maslin-Prothero S E 1994 Race and policy. In: Gough P, Maslin-Prothero S E, Masterson A (eds) Nursing and social policy: care in context. Butterworth-Heinemann, Oxford

Morton-Williams J, Berthoud R 1971 Nurses attitude survey. Social Community Planning Research, London

Nazroo J 1997 The health of Britain's ethnic minorities. Policy Studies Institute, London

OED 1987, OUP, London

Sly F, Murphy P, Theodossiou I 1997 Women in the labour market: results from the spring 1996 labour force survey. Labour Market Trends (March):91–113

Thatcher M 1978 Community Care (12 April)

Vogel L 1983 Marxism and the oppression of women: toward a unitary theory. Rutgers University Press, New Brunswick, NJ

Walby S 1990 Theorising patriarchy. Basil Blackwell, Oxford

Wollstonecraft M 1792 A vindication of the rights of woman.

Wisniewski D (ed) 1997 Annual abstract of statistics. No 133. Stationery Office, London

3

The role of political parties

John Dearlove and Paul Taggart

INTRODUCTION

New Labour swept into power in the general election of 1997 with an overall majority of 179. The resurgence of New Labour confounded those who had been writing off the Labour Party and marked the end of a period of prolonged Conservative government. In recent years, all the major parties have undergone some fundamental changes. In order to secure votes, Labour has become a 'catch-all' centrist party geared to securing votes at the expense of ideology. The Conservatives, under Margaret Thatcher, discovered a radicalism that was certainly not conservative and although it was the Conservative Party which took Britain into Europe, it has increasingly moved towards a Eurosceptic position. The Liberal Democrats, instead of maintaining their traditional distance from both the major parties, are now co-operating with the new Labour government. The electorate has also changed and is now far more fickle in its support for the parties at the polls.

What has not changed, however, is the central role which political parties play within the British system of democracy. That is why it is absolutely vital that you are equipped to understand what political parties are and how they function so that you can appreciate why they have had to change in order to survive in a social and economic environment that is itself changing.

Britain enjoys a system of representative democracy, a system of governance in which citizens take no direct part in governmental decision making but instead elect representatives to govern over them and make public policy on a host of matters from economy to environment, warfare to welfare. For example, the provision of health care in Britain, unlike the provision of such things as clothes and food where the market system is of central importance, is almost entirely organized and provided for by the state out of the public purse and on the basis of policies determined by the government. It is not surprising, therefore, that health is one of the most contentious issues in British party politics, with all parties claiming that the National Health Service is safe in their hands whilst they continue to push different policies with respect to its organization and funding. The NHS (Britain's largest employer with well over 1 million workers, half of whom are nurses) costs some £40 billion to run and absorbs about 15% of all public expenditure. It is under constant pressure to do more with less, precisely because parties are themselves under pressure at the polls to keep down the level of taxation because they believe that high taxes will cost them votes. Within a representative democracy, critical decisions about health care are made by elected politicians in government, and health is invariably an important issue in general elections.

Political parties put up candidates to compete in elections in order to have their candidates elected as representatives to the House of Commons in the hope that they will secure a majority of seats so as to be able to go on to form a government. Elections link the governors to the governed and enable us, the people, to choose our political leaders and hold them to account for their conduct. Political parties in combination with free and fair elections are vital in securing representative and responsible government, the very essence of democracy. It is worrying therefore that many commentators suggest that British parties are far from healthy and that this is either a symptom or a cause of the weakening of democracy in Britain.

Throughout this chapter, and in order to help you understand the part played by political parties within the British system of democracy, we examine a number of different models of parties and party systems. We explore the model of responsible party government and the argument about adversary party politics. We assess the evidence in order to help you decide whether Britain is a multi-party system, a two-party system, or a system where one party has tended to be dominant. We also look at the argument about the decline of the political party. Finally we conclude by offering our assessment as to whether we enjoy a system that offers both representative and responsible government.

While political parties and party systems are clearly related they are not the same thing, and so it is important that you recognize the different processes that affect parties and party systems. Political parties are voluntary organizations that have an independent life each from the other. They draw on different electoral constituencies; are organized in different ways; and, most obviously, are grounded in different ideological traditions. Political parties are the constituent parts of the party system but the system is, by definition, something that is more than just the sum of the parties. The party system, defined here as the relationship between parties, has properties that go beyond the political parties themselves. It creates its own dynamic, and this means that we need to consider the parties together as they interact, as well as separately as organizations in their own right.

THE DEVELOPMENT OF POLITICAL PARTIES AND THE PARTY SYSTEM

Britain is often portrayed as the classic example of a two-party system but it is important to recognize that many more parties exist, some of which are represented in the House of Commons. After the 1997 general election there were 10 different parties represented in the House of Commons, with 75 MPs from the minor parties. New Labour may have won a landslide of seats but its share of the vote was lower than it had achieved in all elections from 1945 to 1966, including the three it actually lost in the 1950s. The Conservative share of the vote was lower than in any parliamentary election since mass franchise. Put another way, the position of the two main parties in the 1990s is very much less secure than it was in the 30 years from 1945, because voters have turned their back on them in favour of rival parties. That said, the election of MPs from third parties has been made difficult by an electoral system that does not deliver seats in proportion to votes. This so-called 'first-past-the-post' system disadvantages parties that do not enjoy a tight geographical base with their voters bunched up in a limited number of constituencies. Whilst the nationalist parties in Wales and in Scotland are well placed to turn votes into seats, Liberal Democrat voters tend to be spread thinly across every constituency.

The Liberal Democrats were born out of a fusion of the Liberal Party, one of the two parties in the 19th-century two-party system, and the Social Democratic Party (SDP), a break-away group from the Labour Party. The perception that the Labour Party was heading left and away from Europe galvanized a group of centrist Labour politicians to form the new party in 1981 (Crewe & King 1995). Their aim was to replace Labour as the alternative to the Conservative Party. In other words, they wanted to realign the party system, replacing competition between Labour and the Conservatives by competition between the SDP and the Conservatives. The failure of the SDP to replace Labour should not necessarily be taken as evidence that realignment is impossible; it happened earlier this century, when the Labour Party replaced the Liberals.

The political parties and the party system have gone through a series of changes in recent decades in Britain. The three major parties have undergone profound shifts in the ideologies that they espouse, and have experienced some serious fluctuations in the support they have received at the polls. These changes are not unusual. Since their foundation over 100 years ago, British political parties have been forced to change both what they do and how they do it in response to larger changes within society and polity. Parties are not just carriers of particular ideologies and aspirations, they are also organizations that need to survive over time.

Without a durable organization it is quite impossible for them to win elections where there is a mass electorate and so be able to put party ideology into governmental practice and public policy. We now take a brief look at the history of British political parties to highlight just how these organizations have had to adapt.

The history of political parties in Britain

The 19th century

In the early part of the 19th century the Conservatives and Liberals emerged within the House of Commons as parliamentary groupings designed to sustain governments in office. These groupings had a limited life outside of the House; they had little need for any formal organization, and so have been described as 'cadre parties'. The fact that the franchise was severely restricted and that only those with money and high social status could possibly become parliamentarians meant that these parties were not interested in collecting members or money, or in organizing voters, since votes could be secured on the basis of patronage and bribery. The franchise was extended from 1832 and as more social groups gradually came to be drawn into politics there was a need to organize masses of voters in order to secure victory.

The 20th century – the rise of the Labour Party

Initially, the electoral battle was fought between Conservatives and Liberals, but the turn of the century saw the formation and then the steady rise of the Labour Party which attracted the support of the newly enfranchised manual working class. This party, like other parties on the left in Europe, drew on the working class as both a basis for branch party membership and as the core of their electoral support. Lacking the resources of the other more established parties they needed a mass membership to supply both the money (through membership dues) and the labour (through the voluntary activities of their members) in order to make the party viable as a fighting force. A mass franchise and secret ballots restricted the scope for corruption and bribery in securing support at the polls and so the other parties had to adapt as well. They were forced to emulate the form of the Labour Party in order to survive and this meant that they too became active in building up their memberships and becoming 'mass parties' with substantial lives outside of parliament.

Postwar developments

In the period after the Second World War, party politics in Britain seemed less ideological and the two major parties came to share a broadly similar agenda that embraced support for the welfare state and the National Health Service, the mixed, but managed, economy and full employment. A period of relative social consensus and harmony based on the long postwar boom meant that the parties basically agreed on the broad parameters of politics and on what to do in office. This growing similarity meant that the parties were less able to differentiate themselves to their potential electorates and so, in the search for votes, they began to appeal to wider constituencies that took them beyond their traditional bases of class support. They became 'catch-all parties'. Party leaders downplayed the importance of ideology and the constraining significance of party members. Interest groups were relied on more heavily for finance. Party leaders also played up their own power and position as the public face of the party in election battles that have become increasingly personalized and presidential.

Historically, the Labour Party has been associated with 'collectivist' ideas, that is ideas that involve the public provision of services in place of market provision, which they see as biased in favour of the better off. For their part, the Conservative Party, although sometimes portrayed as lacking any ideology, has consistently built itself around the defence of order and stability. This has meant that they have, on the one hand, attacked socialism as both inefficient and as destructive of that stability, and on the other they have championed the virtues of the market as an effective alternative to state planning. The Liberal Party played a key role in developing the idea of the welfare state at the turn of the 20th century, although it was the Labour government of 1945 that was the architect of the National Health Service. As the state became more involved in providing health care and there was money available consequent upon economic growth, there was a general consensus between the parties to support and expand the health service. But when the boom ended in the 1970s, British politics became far less consensual and the NHS was drawn into party political battles. The ideas of the New Right, an ideology that celebrated the virtues of the market and attacked state provision and taxation, permeated the Conservative Party and moved it to the right. The Labour Party responded by rediscovering old ideological roots in socialism on the left. The election of Margaret Thatcher in 1979 was seen as an attack on the very idea of the public provision of many services, including health. Labour's response was to champion its defence of the NHS. It is no coincidence that in various opinion polls of nurses, the Labour Party has consistently been seen as the party most associated with the defence of the NHS. For example, in a poll of nurses conducted for the *Nursing Times* before the 1997 election, 32% trusted Labour with the NHS compared to only 5% who trusted the Conservatives (Nursing Times 1997).

At the same time as party politics was polarizing, parties themselves and the very process of electoral and parliamentary politics came under attack from new social movements. These movements, including the feminist movement, the environmental movement and the peace movement, rejected established modes of political action and advocated direct action and the politics of protest.

Trade unions

It is against this historical and political background that we need to understand the recent changes that have taken place in British political parties. The changes within the Labour Party which culminated in Blair's 1997 election victory go beyond Blair and back to the leadership of Neil Kinnock and John Smith. After its defeat in the 1983 election when the Labour Party took a strong left-wing position, the party gradually changed both its policies and the way it was organized in order to maximize support from outside its traditional base in the working class. The party organization changed in the emphasis given to the power of the trade unions.

The power of the unions had been a key issue in British politics in the 1970s and the Conservative government had played on a distrust of unions by introducing a series of legislative bills to curb their power. After the 1983 defeat, Neil Kinnock saw the need to break the link between Labour and the unions. Traditionally, Labour was a party that had been formed by the trade unions to put working class representatives into the Commons, and the unions have continued to be the major funders of the party. For a period, this gave certain sorts of unions access to power through the Labour Party and may explain why other sectors have felt themselves excluded.

Unions and workforces not organized in the manner of traditional heavy industry have felt themselves under-represented. Nursing is one such case; the nature of its representation through unions may explain why nurses are seen as not having access to power through the Labour Party. Looking at the representation of nurses it is clear that a number of factors are at play here. First, the Labour Party was formed by unions representing men in the traditional heavy industries of mining and manufacture and this gave those unions an insider status of power that made them resistant to any newcomers. Second, the Royal College of Nursing (RCN), formed by matrons in 1916, did not register as a union until 1977. It has consistently adopted a no-strike policy and has chosen neither to affiliate to the Trades Union Congress (the national organization for unions in Britain) nor to tie itself into the party political battle. Instead the RCN has chosen to see itself as a professional organization rather than as a traditional trade union. Third, about half of all nurses have been organized into rival trade unions, most notably COSHE and NUPE, and this has meant that there has never been one organization to articulate the demands of nurses in the political process. Only since the amalgamation of the nursing unions of COSHE and NUPE into UNISON in 1993 as the largest union in Britain, with a membership of 1.4 million, has there opened up the prospect of nurses securing more of an impact on the policy process.

To restrict the power of the unions at the Labour Party Conference, which has always been the ultimate decision making body for Labour, John Smith, who led the party between 1992 and 1996, introduced the idea of 'one member one vote'. This had the effect of reducing the power of the union block vote whereby the unions had votes at conference in proportion to their membership. This change was voted through the party's conference. Tony Blair became leader following John Smith's sudden death in 1996. Under Tony Blair, New Labour has sought to secure a mass membership of individuals to provide money and volunteers and to break the hold of the unions. That said, wary of the experience of extremist constituency activism in the 1980s, the leadership of the party wanted a passive membership of supporters rather than an active membership of demanding extremists. This aspiration to become a mass membership party needs to be evaluated against the falling membership of the Labour Party from a high of about 1 million in 1952 down to about 0.25 million in the 1970s and 1980s. Blair has publicly committed the party to a membership of 0.5 million by the year 2001, but this looks to be optimistic.

Another controversial change effected by Labour was the introduction of all-women short lists in certain constituencies. Short lists are the lists of individuals who want to become candidates at a general election, with local parties choosing one from the list to serve as their prospective parliamentary candidate at a general election. By ensuring that women were chosen as candidates in certain seats the Labour Party was attempting to ensure that more women became MPs, so making the House of Commons less of an all-male club. After the 1992 election just 9% of the House of Commons were women but after the 1997 election this figure had increased to 18%, with 101 of the 119 women MPs being representatives of Labour.

For their part, the Conservative Party have felt little need to agonize about their form of organization precisely because this century has belonged to them. Constitutionally and legally there is no single body known as the Conservative Party. There are three separate organizations; the parliamentary party, the extra-parliamentary National Union of Conservative Associations, and the professional staff in Central Office. Each of the three organizations has different but overlapping responsibilities; all have their own separate hierarchy; and so it is quite possible for the three separate organizations to pursue different strategies and competing priorities. None of this mattered when the party was assured of electoral success but the electoral disaster of 1997 forced them to give serious thought to both their ideology and their organization. Their active membership had fallen from almost 2.5 million in 1953 to about 0.25 million by 1997, the majority of whom were over 65 years old. The fact that the Conservative Party had long been a leadership-dominated, top-down party was likely to do little to encourage more membership in an age when those joining parties were keen to have an impact. Not surprisingly, William Hague, who took over the leadership of the Conservative Party in 1997, expressed a concern to 'democratise' the party (Hague 1997) and encouraged a situation when ordinary members would have a say in choosing the leader. In other words, Hague decided that members of the Conservative Party should be consulted to a much greater extent on the way in which the party is run.

RESPONSIBLE PARTY GOVERNMENT

If one of the functions of a political party is to serve as a link between the governors and the governed, then it is vital that parties are able and willing to effect that link and represent us responsibly. This means that parties can be judged as valuable within a democracy to the extent that they are able to represent the electorate and are capable of delivering the policies they promise when they seek our votes at general elections.

The model of responsible party government

The model of 'responsible party government' sets down the conditions that need to be met if it is to be the case that parties shape up and actually do work to make for a system of governmental responsibility to us, the electors. In bald terms, the model makes a number of assumptions as to what is needed of parties and the system of electoral competition if we are to secure responsible government. The model assumes that there is a two-party system sustained by regular free and fair elections. These two parties are in close competition, each with the other, to form a government, and therefore they have to be sensitive to changes in what the electorate want of government. The two parties compete by offering themselves up to the electorate on the basis of election manifestos which are composed of a series of policy promises that comprise a policy package, or programme, that may reflect either ideology or a certain approach to government. For their part, individual voters decide which party to support on the basis of the issues and what the parties have to offer in their programmes. At a general election one party will usually be successful in winning a clear majority of seats in the House of Commons so that it will then be able to form the government, with a mandate to implement the programme of policy promises contained in their election manifesto. The party which loses the election has the important function of opposition in order to prevent the governing party from resting on its laurels and being insensitive to changes in public opinion at the same time as the opposition party will be revising its own stance on policies with a view to developing a programme that will prove to be more popular at the next election. The final assumption of the model of 'responsible party government' is that the parties are disciplined organizations so that MPs have a clear obligation to put the party line before their own consciences.

Does the model work?

The model of responsible party government is just that, a model. It is an idealised conception as to how a party system *should* work if responsibility to electors is to be assured. But does the British party system actually work like this? Let us examine the 'fit' between the assumptions in the model and the reality of party and electoral practice with respect to three broad areas.

First, and with respect to the voters, do voters actually choose a party on the basis of the issues and the programme offered or is there a better explanation for the factors behind our electoral choices? Second, and with respect to the behaviour of the parties in the House of Commons, are the parties disciplined teams so that party leaders can rely on solid support in order to secure the legislation needed to vote through the manifesto programmes? And third, and fundamentally, do governments actually deliver on their electoral promises?

The voters – how do they make their choices?

Do voters actually choose a party on the basis of the issues and the programmes offered? There are many different, and competing, explanations of why people vote the way they do. In the 1960s, Butler & Stokes (1969) suggested that voters did not so much *choose* a party and a programme of policies as *identify* with a party on the basis of attachments that were formed in early life as a result of socialization in the home. More than this, they further suggested that voters were often ignorant of the issues and may well have voted for a party not because of its policies but in spite of them. Butler & Stokes were sensitive to the importance of class in British politics. They detected a close tie-up between class and party: the middle class tended to support the Conservative Party just as the working class supported and identified with the Labour Party. Butler & Stokes saw in this tie-up an explanation for voting behaviour itself because it was rather assumed that each party would work for the interests of the class that supported it. They would not have been surprised to find out that in a 1992 poll of nurses the senior nurses, in managerial positions, were more likely to vote Conservative than their junior colleagues (Nursing Times 1992).

In the 1970s, surveys of voters suggested that the tie-up between class and party was very much less tight than once was the case and that this, together with the decline in the attachment of voters to the two major parties, was opening up electoral space. In effect, the decline in class voting and the decline in attachments to parties created a volatile situation in which voters were free to choose on the issues in a fairly rational and self-interested manner. Voters were seen as political consumers, using their votes as kind of political money in order to purchase that package of policies which best secured their interests. This view of how voters decided offered support for one of the conditions central to the model of 'responsible party government': voters were choosing on the basis of the issues.

Särlvik & Crewe's analysis of the 1979 general election (Särlvik & Crewe 1983) was clear in arguing that the Conservatives won because the majority of the electorate preferred the policies of the Conservatives to those of tired and out-of-date old Labour. That said, the subsequent victories of the Conservatives in 1982, 1987 and 1992 cannot be explained simply as a result of the popularity of the party's policies because the electorate never fully embraced Thatcherite values, being more centrist in their stance to most policy issues. The Conservative dominance of electoral politics in the 1980s was less a function of policies and issues and more a function of a divided opposition vote between Labour and the Liberal Democrats. Also, few were attracted to a Labour Party that lacked unity and was seen as too extreme in its policy positions.

Three factors go some way towards explaining the landslide victory of New Labour in 1997. Firstly, there was a widespread sentiment that it was 'time for a change'. Secondly, the Conservative government was riddled with internal conflicts, had been tainted by allegations of 'sleaze' and as a consequence its competence was being questioned. Finally, there was a new found unity and moderation of Labour under the charismatic leadership of Tony Blair. However, other issues were also significant. For example, opinion polls during the course of the campaign showed that health care was the single most important issue in helping people to decide which party to vote for, with 68% of the electorate viewing the issue in these terms on the very eve of the election (MORI 1997). More than this, Labour was seen as the party which had the best policies on health care, just as it was in front on a number of other issues that were of importance to the electorate, including education, unemployment, pensions and housing. Issues may never have quite the importance that they should have according to the model of responsible party government. This is because the voting decision is the result of a complex number of considerations, but issues are by no means irrelevant and elections do enable us, the voters, to pass a rough judgement on the parties and on the programmes that are set before us.

The parties – party discipline

Are the parties disciplined teams so that party leaders can

rely on support to secure the legislation needed to vote through the manifesto programmes? The importance of factional or internal party conflict has been to the fore in both Labour and Conservative parties in the past 2 decades. In the Labour Party, under the leadership of Neil Kinnock, there were bitter conflicts between the left of the party and its centre as the party attempted to expel left-wing extremists in the mid-1980s. In the 1990s, the Conservative Party was riven with factional conflicts as the issue of European integration polarized MPs and led to some rebels being thrown out of the parliamentary party for not toeing the party line. Such internal conflict was not new. During the period of Thatcher's leadership a line had been driven between the one nation 'Wets' and the 'Dries'. The 'Wets' were broadly in support of maintaining levels of social spending whereas the 'Dries' were advocates of drastic reduction in support for the welfare state as they applauded the virtues of the market and all things private.

Even when parties are not riven by open conflicts, it is still the case that they are composed of very different groups of MPs and that below the surface there is always a constant struggle for control of the heart and soul of any party. Often these conflicts become most apparent when there is the possibility of a change of leader. For in these times there is an opportunity for groups that have felt excluded to try and place one of 'their own' in power. Rose suggested in 1964 that the Conservative Party was given to conflict between tendencies while the Labour Party was given to factional conflict. He differentiated these two by suggesting that tendencies were constant streams of thought that, over time, attracted different party members to them, whereas factions were more constant groups of members with similar views. The recent history of the two major parties may well dispel Rose's idea of the Conservative Party being free of faction, but it does not disguise the fact that the internal life of political parties is always one of conflict, compromise, and co-operation between party members with very different views.

The effect of this conflict within parties is that they can never be quite sure that they will not face a rebellion from the back-benches of their own party. Norton (1997) has done extensive work on the nature of back-bench rebellion and Table 3.1 shows the extent of dissent in the Commons. The table illustrates the fact that there has been a significant growth in the tendency for MPs to vote against the party line since the 1970s. The reality is that while MPs still depend on their party for election, that their party cannot always depend on them for support in the Commons.

Table 3.1 House of Commons votes and the extent of dissent, 1945–1997 (data from Norton 1997)

Parliament	Number of divisions witnessing dissenting votes		Number of divisions witnessing dissenting votes expressed as % of all divisions
	Labour	**Conservative**	
1945–50	79	27	7.0
1950–51	5	2	2.5
1951–55	17	11	3.0
1955–59	10	12	2.0
1959–64	26	120	13.5
1964–66	1	1	0.5
1966–70	109	41	9.5
1970–74	34	204	20
1974	8	21	23
1974–79	309	240	28
1979–83	161	158	19
1983–87	83	202	22
1987–92	137	199	19
1992–97	143	170	20.5

The government – keeping election promises

Finally, in our assessment of the model of responsible party government, we ask whether governments actually deliver their election promises. This is the nub of the matter. Many major policies have been introduced without them ever having been set before the electorate for approval or disapproval. More than this, we all know that the very stuff of electoral competition revolves around the issue of U-turns and broken promises, with governments confessing (but excusing and explaining) the gap between election promise and ruling performance with talk about being blown off course by events beyond their control. Careful work by Hofferbert & Budge (1992, p. 151) found that 'what governments do relates broadly either to their manifesto emphases or to their long-standing ideological commitments', although they go on to say that 'Labour manifesto commitments are a bad indicator of what they will do in government'.

Health care issues With respect to the health care issue in the 1997 election, what becomes clear is that there was a great deal of policy consensus between the parties. All parties were committed to the 'purchaser–provider split', to the concept of a primary care led NHS and to the importance of private capital being used to fund the building of NHS hospitals. This consensus makes it difficult for voters to choose between parties. We can tease out some specific promises that Labour made, such as their commitment to increase expenditure on patient care through reducing expenditure on bureaucracy and red tape; their concern to abolish the internal market in the NHS whilst retaining the idea of the purchaser–provider split; and their concern to abolish GP fundholding. Looking at the White Paper *The new NHS: modern, dependable* (NHS 1997), produced by the Labour

Party after its electoral victory, it is already clear that the government is keen to implement its promises. For example, it is looking to save some £1 billion on bureaucracy over the lifetime of the Parliament, although it is vague as to how this will be accomplished, and it talks about 'going beyond' GP fundholding rather than abolishing it altogether. Just looking at a government White Paper is, of course, not the same as seeing whether a promise is being delivered, but it does give us some idea as to whether a party in government is actually trying to follow through on its election promises. Whether these promises and plans come to fruition remains to be seen.

The model of responsible party government has never been a close description of the reality of party politics in Britain but elements of political practice have come close, and it does provide a set of benchmark standards from which to assess the responsibility of British party politics. Other perspectives on party politics in Britain have been very much more critical of the practice of that politics, none more so than the model of 'adversary party politics' that came to the fore in the 1970s, turning many of the responsible party government perspectives on their heads.

ADVERSARY PARTY POLITICS

The importance of alternation between responsible parties is the central feature of the responsible party government model. This model is clearly very dependent on the nature of British politics, as it is one of the effects of the British electoral system to reinforce the two-party nature of the House of Commons. It is difficult for new, smaller parties to break through unless they have a regional concentration in their vote as is the case with nationalist parties in Scotland and

Wales. The electoral system also tends to magnify the position of the winning party in the House of Commons, giving them seats out of proportion to their votes in the country. These two facts combined mean that the party system in Parliament is given to alternation between the two dominant parties with each having a relatively strong hold on power when in office in what is a very centralized system.

This situation has led to the suggestion that British party politics is more adversarial than responsible. In contrast to the responsible party government model, then, the adversarial party politics model suggests that politics is damaged by the constant alternation between parties.

The adversary party politics thesis emerged during the 1970s (Finer 1975). At this time there were fundamental conflicts between the parties concerning issues of economic and social policy. The emergence of Margaret Thatcher as leader of the Conservative Party in 1974 presaged a period of ideological conflict and conviction politics. The election of the 1979 Thatcher government had two effects. It changed the Conservative Party by pushing it towards a more pro-market, rolling back the state position on the right of the ideological spectrum. The shift away from the centre ground on the part of the Conservatives also had the effect of forcing Labour into a more confrontational position on the left of British politics. British party politics was polarized. Adversarial politics was seen as problematic, partly because it was a polarized and confrontational politics but also because it was seen as involving policy reversals that failed to provide the kind of policy continuity that was seen as so important in securing Britain's economic success. Gamble & Walkland (1984, p. 174), in their study *The British party system and economic policy: 1945–1983*, were concerned to see how many economic policies were actually reversed by an incoming government over the period between 1960 and 1981. They claim that the adversary party politics thesis 'generalises from a few instances to the whole of economic policy' and that it fails to recognize the need to distinguish between foreign economic policy, stabilization policy, and industrial and commercial policy. According to Gamble & Walkland (1984, p. 176), 'the evidence that there have been significant discontinuities in economic policy-making caused by the adversary positions adopted by the parties seems to be limited to industrial policy'. The 'major issues of foreign economic policy have been marked by continuity'. Although membership of the European Community hovered on the edge of becoming subject to adversary party politics, it never did, and the divisions within the parties have continued to be of more significance than the differences between the two main parties. With respect to stabilization policy, 'the evidence for continuity is rather more plain than the evidence for discontinuity'.

Under-representation

The adversary nature of the party system has also been seen as one of the reasons for the under-representation of certain social groups. If the model assumes alternation between two parties, then this limits the options for new parties. If, in addition to this, the existing parties restrict access to certain groups, then the problem is compounded. Norris & Lovenduski (1995), in writing about the representation of women, have stressed the role that institutional factors have played in the under-representation of women in the British parties. They stress that there are factors determining who stands and factors determining whether they are successful. If we simply look at the representation of nurses as parliamentary candidates in the last three elections, it becomes clear that the winning of seats by nurses is not simply related to the number contesting seats. The 1997 election yielded two nurses as MPs while there were seven other unsuccessful parliamentary candidates. In 1992 success was less but there were 12 nursing candidates. In 1987 there were only six nurses standing. The success of Ann Keen and Laura Moffat in 1997 may owe much to the fact that of the nine candidates, they were the only two Labour candidates, and therefore their success owed as much to Labour's national success as to their persistence. Many of the other candidates were contesting elections in regions where their party had little hope of success. The adversary politics thesis has always tended to be something of a partisan and political perspective. It was central to the position of the SDP and the Liberal Democrats, who were critical of both left and right at the same time as the electoral system excluded them from their 'fair' share of seats in the Commons. The fact that Thatcher was ousted from power in 1990 led to a moderation of conservatism at the same time as Labour moved to the centre in order to garner votes in ways that makes the adversary thesis now look rather dated as a description of contemporary party politics. That said, the perspective of the Conservatives after their 1997 election defeat, and the possibility of division within the Labour government should remind us that it is always possible for party politics to have an ugly adversarial and polarized aspect.

ONE PARTY DOMINANCE

The Conservative Party

The period 1979–1997 represented, for many, the transformation of British party politics into Conservative Party politics. The success of the Conservatives in four successive elections (1979, 1983, 1987 and 1992), under Margaret Thatcher and John Major, meant that some people declared that the era of competitive party politics was over. This was called the 'Japanization' of British politics because Britain was, it was argued, coming to resemble Japanese politics which has long been dominated by a single party (Margetts & Smyth 1994). Conservative dominance of British party politics was, however, not a new suggestion. Gamble (1974) suggested in *The Conservative nation* that the party's ability to construct itself around the goal of power meant that it was a different type of party to its more ideologically-driven competitors in Britain and a far more successful one to boot. If we consider that the Conservative Party has been in government for 68 of the 98 years of the 20th century, then the Conservative dominance between 1979 and 1997 appears less exceptional. Seldon & Ball (1994) have gone so far as to characterize the 20th century as the 'Conservative century'.

The period of Conservative domination came to an end in May 1997 with the election of New Labour under Tony Blair. The period prior to the Conservative defeat, and especially the latter period of John Major's administration, was marked by a high degree of factional conflict within the party. That conflict was primarily around the issue of European integration which ran, like a fault line, through the Conservative Party and its ideology. Conservative MPs saw in the European issue a conflict between the traditional nationalism of the Conservative Party which would lead them to oppose the extension of European integration, and the commitment to the free market and its internationalizing potential which would lead them to support further European integration. The intensification of factional conflict led Ted Heath, the former Conservative prime minister, to describe the Eurosceptics as a 'party within a party'. In some ways, divisions within the Conservative Party meant that the party itself became a kind of party system in its own right; a substitute for the wider party system where Labour was so weak. Put another way, effective opposition occurred within the Conservative Party, and this factional conflict replaced the 'normal' pattern of party conflict.

The Labour Party

At the same time as the Conservative Party was becoming divided over Europe, the Labour Party was undergoing drastic change. In ideological terms, it had moved towards a much more centrist position. It had abandoned its commitment to Clause IV, that part of the Labour Party constitution that committed the party to the nationalization of industry and socialism itself. There was a heavy symbolism to the dropping of Clause IV, which had been seen by the left wing of the party as a touchstone of its socialist ideology. With the abandonment of Clause IV the party had 'modernized' itself to bring itself in line with its social democratic sister parties in other parts of Europe and had moved towards the centre of British politics.

It is clear that prolonged periods of domination by one party lead to a very different type of party system. In contrast to the adversarial model in which the parties construct themselves as mirror images of each other, under one party dominance the dominant party comes under intense internal pressure, while the other parties face intense external pressure to change in order to break the hold of the dominant party. We see in the 1997 election both the breaking of the dominance of one party but also the clear effect of a sustained period in government by one party in that both major parties look significantly different than they appeared in 1979.

MULTI-PARTY POLITICS

Throughout this chapter we have addressed the issue of whether Britain is really a two-party system. Looking at the one party thesis is one end of the spectrum, but there are also perspectives and good reasons why we can describe Britain, at the other end of the spectrum, as having multi-party politics. In the 1970s and early 1980s there was a school of thought that Britain had become a multi-party system as this period saw the growth in strength of regional parties in Scotland and Wales and the arrival of the SDP (Drucker 1979). While the subsequent collapse of the SDP undermined the argument that this period saw something qualitatively new emerge, there are long-term trends in the support for the parties that give credence to the idea that, at some level, Britain has multi-party politics.

Regional influences

Changes in electoral behaviour since the Second World War have meant that while at a national level the composition of the House of Commons remains broadly similar, at a more regional level the parties have come to occupy very different positions in different parts of Britain. The two key changes are the collapse of the Conservative Party in Scotland, effectively making much of Scotland a two-party system with competition being between the Labour Party and the Scottish National Party. The second regional change has been the regionalization of the support for the Liberal Democrats. Their heartland has become the south-west of England. The third change has been the decline of the Labour vote in the south of England generally. This is shown by the figures in Table 3.2.

Table 3.2 Regional distribution of the British vote, 1955 and 1992 (Norris 1997, p. 130)

	1955	1992	Change	1955	1992	Change	1955	1992	Change
	Con	Con		Lab	Lab		Lib	LibDem	
South-West	52	47	−5	39	20	−19	9	31	22
South-East	58	54	−14	39	21	−18	2	23	21
East Anglia	52	51	−1	47	29	−18	1	19	18
Greater London	54	44	−10	51	38	−13	2	15	13
West Midlands	50	44	−7	48	40	−8	2	15	13
East Midlands	47	46	−1	51	38	−13	1	15	14
Wales	31	28	−3	60	49	−11	4	13	9
Yorkshire and Humberside	45	36	−9	53	46	−6	2	16	14
North	43	33	−10	56	51	−5	4	16	12
North-West	53	37	−16	46	46	1	1	16	15
Scotland	51	24	−27	46	40	−6	1	13	12
Britain	51	41	−10	48	37	−11	2	18	15

Parliament

Parliament has not been immune to these changes because there has been an increase in the number of parties represented in the House of Commons. Both Conservative and Labour governments have increasingly relied on the support of other smaller parties in Parliament to sustain them with a majority. Sometimes this arrangement has been formalized, as in the case of the 'Lib–Lab' pact (March 1977 to May 1979), when the Liberal Party supported the Labour government under James Callaghan. At other times the cooperation has been de facto, as with the Northern Irish Unionist parties' support for the Conservative government in the latter part of John Major's administration.

Local government

Cooperation between parties is not confined to the national level. Indeed it is in the local government sector that we see the most extensive cooperation and the strongest evidence of real multi-party politics. The two major parties have remained strong in London and the Metropolitan borough seats but between 1973 and 1992 they won three-quarters of English shire county seats, roughly two-thirds of the seats in the Scottish regional and district councils and only half of Welsh county and district seats (Norris 1997, pp. 48–49). This has forced a large number of local government administrations to form coalitions across party lines.

The European Union

At a rather different level, the growing importance of the European Union provides another arena for party competition. It must be admitted that scope for competition is rather weak as the European Parliament, whose members are directly elected, is the weakest EU institution. None the less, it is becoming clear that the cooperation between similar parties in different countries is having an effect on individual parties and there is the potential for something like a wider European party system to emerge should the role of the European Parliament be strengthened. For Britain, a party system more integrated (at least at one level) with other European party systems necessarily means a more multi-party system, as all the countries except Britain have multi-party systems. The competition for national office is the most important arena for understanding the British party system, but this is not the same as saying that there are no other areas we need to explore to capture the full scope of the party system. A look beyond the walls of Westminster, to regional trends within the national vote, to local government and to the European Union gives strong evidence that there are good reasons for considering some aspects of the British party system as characterized by multi-party politics.

THE DECLINE OF PARTY AND THE RISE OF ANTI-PARTY SENTIMENT

In recent years, many people have challenged the relevance of political parties. Those challenges have not been confined to Britain; parties around the world have also come under attack, with party systems in countries as diverse as Italy, Japan and Canada undergoing major changes. We have already seen that the emergence of new political actors in the form of the new social movements has led to the rejection of party politics. This change on the part of political actors has been matched by an increasing sensitivity on the part of academic observers to the issue of the decline of party and the rise of anti-party sentiment (Daalder 1992, Poguntke 1996).

Poguntke (1996) suggests that we need to look at four different factors in order to assess whether parties are in decline in any country:

- First, he suggests that we need to look at voter turnout at elections. Simply, this is the idea that if people are not bothering to turn out to vote then it may reflect their disenchantment with the parties on offer at the election.

- Second, he suggests that we should consider whether voters are becoming less attached and committed to the mainstream parties.

- Third, we need to look at whether fewer people are becoming members of parties.

• And finally, he suggests that we should consider whether there has been a growth in the number of 'anti-party parties', parties which base their appeal on their rejection of the dominant pattern of party politics.

Let us see the facts with respect to these four points.

Voter turnout. Has electoral turnout declined in Britain? In 1950, turnout was 84% but by 1997 turnout had fallen to a record postwar low of 71% as 12 million voters chose to stay at home.

Voter commitment. Are voters are becoming less attached and committed to the mainstream parties? Table 3.3 shows clearly that, whilst in 1951 the two main parties between them could count on 97% of the vote, by the mid-1970s this was down to 75% and has never really recovered.

Views of nurses. It is striking that nurses have both reflected this trend and, at times, taken it further. In a poll of nurses before the 1997 election, 41% of nurses said that they would trust none of the existing parties with the NHS – 18% said the same before the 1992 election (Nursing Times 1997). Among those nurses who do support a particular party the period between 1992 and 1997 saw a steep rise in support for Labour and a decline in Conservative support (see Table 3.4). While voting nurses have clearly favoured Labour in recent years, the biggest change is the increase in opting out of party politics, in line with many in the general population.

Party membership. Are fewer people becoming members of parties? As we have already seen, in the mid-1950s the Conservative Party claimed a membership of 2.8 million

Table 3.3 Conservative and Labour shares of the vote, 1945–97 (*Nursing Times* 25 March 1992 and 29 January 1997)

Election	Conservative	Labour	Combined
1945	40	48	88
1950	43	46	89
1951	48	49	97
1955	50	46	96
1959	49	44	93
1964	43	44	87
1966	42	48	90
1970	46	43	89
1974 (February)	38	37	75
1974 (October)	36	39	75
1979	44	37	81
1983	42	28	70
1987	42	31	73
1992	42	34	76
1997	31	44	75

Table 3.4 Voting intentions of nurses in pre-election polls (*Nursing Times* 25 March 1992 and 29 January 1997)

	1977 (%)	1992 (%)
Labour	70	43
Conservative	16	33
LibDem	11	20
Other	3	4

and Labour a membership of just over one million but by the 1990s the Conservative membership had fallen three quarters of a million and Labour could claim little more than 400 000.

'Anti-party parties'. Has there been a growth in the number of 'anti-party parties' in Britain? In 1997 there were more candidates standing in the general election than ever before (3717). Most of the fringe parties had their moment of glory but lost their deposits. On the one hand we have seen broad-based parties such as the Green Party appearing on the political map. These sorts of parties have a broad agenda and have tried to organize themselves in a way that is deliberately different to the mainstream parties but in doing so have restricted their effectiveness and have never really achieved representation in the House of Commons. On the other hand there has also been a rise in single-issue based parties and candidates such as the Referendum Party. This highly Eurosceptic party, led by a millionaire, the late Sir James Goldsmith, attained 3% of the vote, but only after spending £20 million or £24.68 per vote. Ironically, the net effect was to let in some more Europhile Labour MPs.

Notwithstanding evidence that supports the view that there has been 'a decline in party', it continues to be the case that political parties survive, though with less support, at the very heart of politics and policy making in Britain. The election of New Labour in 1997, although based on 44% of the voters and 31% of the electorate, still came to power with the intention of enacting some wide-ranging reforms, not the least of which were the plans for the health service.

CONCLUSION: REPRESENTATIVE AND RESPONSIBLE GOVERNMENT?

In our introduction we highlighted the importance of political parties providing for representative and responsible government. All of the perspectives we have looked at touch on these matters. If party practice was in accord with the essentials of the model of 'responsible party government' then we could feel comfortable with our system of democracy. If practice was more at one with the adversary party politics model or we were truly stuck with a system of one-party dominance, then any good democrat would have cause for concern. Such a person might also be concerned at the extent to which the two main parties still dominate the composition of the House of Commons. Although about 25% of the electorate regularly vote for third parties, those parties fail to secure much more than 10% of the seats in the Commons. This failure of our electoral system to deliver seats in the Commons in proportion to votes in the country highlights the possibility of a tension between the twin goals of representation and responsibility where there is always going to be the necessity for some kind of trade-off. The great virtue of two-party politics, with one party in government, is that it enables us, the voters, to pass rough but clear judgements at the polls. The absence of coalition government means that it is always obvious which party has been in government at the same time as there is just one opposition party available to replace the old government. But more than this, the party system does not have to be frozen. In the 20th century Liberals were replaced by Labour, and in the 1980s the SDP-Liberal Alliance came close to replacing Labour. In this kind of party and electoral situation, holding a government responsible to the people at an election is to the fore even though it may mean that third parties are not 'fairly' represented in the Commons in proportion to their votes in the country. In a word, responsibility is at a premium over representation within our system of democracy.

■ QUESTIONS FOR DISCUSSION

- To what extent can Britain be described as a two-party system?
- Explore the case for proportional representation.

■ **QUESTIONS FOR DISCUSSION** (*cont'd*)

- What do you understand by adversary party politics and what are its effects?
- What strategy should opposition parties adopt in order to win elections?
- When you vote, do you consider the programmes of the parties and vote on the issues?
- What evidence would you put forward to suggest that Britain is either a one-party or a multi-party system?

FURTHER READING

Ball A 1987 British political parties: the emergence of a modern party system. Macmillan, Basingstoke

This book provides an historical overview of the development of the parties since 1867.

Butler D, Stokes D 1969 Political change in Britain. Macmillan, London

A classic study of voting behaviour which drew heavily on the experience of explaining voting behaviour in the USA and which put forward the idea of 'party identification' as the key to understanding British voting.

Crewe I, King A 1995 SDP: The birth, life and death of the Social Democratic Party. Oxford University Press, Oxford

This definitive volume charts the history of the SDP and is written by two academics who were involved in advising the fledgling party.

Finer S E (ed) 1975 Adversary politics and electoral reform. Anthony Wigram, London

This is a classic statement of the adversary politics thesis, together with a plea for electoral reform.

Margetts H, Smyth G (eds) 1994 Turning Japanese? Britain with a permanent party of government. Lawrence and Wishart, London

Written before the election of New Labour and so now rather dated, but the essays convey something of the air of disillusionment that pervaded British politics after four terms of Conservative government.

Maor M 1997 Political parties and party systems: comparative approaches and the British experience. Routledge, London

Unusually for a book on British political parties, this author takes a comparative approach and looks at Britain using perspectives and theories that apply to parties elsewhere in the world.

Norris P 1997 Electoral change since 1945. Blackwell, Oxford

This book provides an accessible and up-to-date guide to voting behaviour in Britain.

Norris P, Lovenduski J 1995 Political recruitment: gender, race and class in the British Parliament. Cambridge University Press, Cambridge

The authors provide a thorough examination of the ways in which the different British parties recruit and select parliamentary politicians, and particularly explores the relative lack of women, black and working-class MPs.

Seyd P, Whiteley P 1992 Labour's grass roots: the politics of party membership. Clarendon Press, Oxford

This book is the result of an extensive survey into the nature of the Labour Party's membership.

Whiteley P, Seyd P, Richardson J 1994 True Blues: the politics of Conservative Party membership. Clarendon Press, Oxford

This book is the result of an extensive survey into the nature of the Conservative Party's membership and is the only up-to-date study of the subject.

REFERENCES

Butler D, Stokes D 1969 Political change in Britain. Macmillan, London

Crewe I, King A 1995 SDP: the birth, life and death of the Social Democratic Party. Oxford University Press, Oxford

Daalder H 1992 A crisis of party. Scandinavian Political Studies 15(4):269–288

Drucker H (ed) 1979 Multi-party Britain. Macmillan, London

Finer S E (ed) 1975 Adversary politics and electoral reform. Anthony Wigram, London

Gamble A 1974 The Conservative nation. Routledge, London

Gamble A, Walkland S 1984 The British party system and economic policy, 1945–1983. Clarendon Press, Oxford

Hague W 1997 Address to Conservative Central Office. 23 July 1997

Hofferbert R I, Budge I 1992 The party mandate and the Westminster model: election programmes and government spending in Britain, 1948–85. British Journal of Political Science 22:151–185

Margetts H, Smyth G (eds) 1994 Turning Japanese? Britain with a permanent party of government. Lawrence and Wishart, London

MORI 1997 British Public Opinion 20(April–June):3–4

NHS 1997 The new NHS: modern, dependable. HMSO, London

Norris P, Lovenduski J 1995 Political recruitment: gender, race and class in the British Parliament. Cambridge University Press, Cambridge

Norton P 1997 Parliamentary oversight. In: Dunleavy P, Gamble A, Holliday I, Peele G (eds) Developments in British politics 5. Macmillan, London

Norris P 1997 Electoral change since 1945. Blackwell, Oxford

Poguntke T 1996 Anti-party sentiment – conceptual thoughts and empirical evidence: explorations into a minefield. European Journal of Political Research 29(3):365–382

Nursing Times 1992 News items. 88(13, 29 January)

Nursing Times 1997 News items. 93(5, 25 March)

Rose R 1964 Parties, factions and tendencies in Britain. Political Studies 12(1):33–46

Särlvick B, Crewe I 1983 Decade of dealignment. Cambridge University Press, Cambridge

Seldon A, Ball S (eds) 1994 Conservative century. Oxford University Press, Oxford

The role of interest groups

Ailsa Cameron

INTRODUCTION

The aim of this chapter is to introduce the reader to the concept of interest groups and their role within the policy making arena. In order to do this I will consider various typologies of interest groups that have been developed by well known political theorists, drawing on examples of groups from within the health policy arena, many of which will already be known to the reader. I will consider the strategies that groups use to influence the formulation of policy and also consider why governments may seek actively to work with these groups.

WHAT IS AN INTEREST GROUP?

It may be tempting to picture our political system narrowly as one defined by rigid structures in which a limited number of political parties seek to win government office in order that they can control the policy making process. In reality, the political system does not begin and end with a general election, nor is it made up only of clearly identified political actors. The system is far more complicated, as previous chapters have indicated.

The democratic political process is continuous, involving constant negotiation and bartering between groups in an attempt to develop and implement government policy. This process, as many theorists have identified (Masterson 1994), brings into play formal mechanisms and actors of government such as government ministers and civil servants. However, it is not just these formal actors who influence the decision making process. Many groups, articulating a variety of interests, will attempt to influence how and what decisions are made at formal and informal levels. These groups are known as interest groups and they are usually made up of persons who share a particular concern and seek to represent that concern within the decision making process. Any study of the political process in Britain would not be complete without an exploration of these groups which appear to have increased their role greatly in recent years.

WHAT MAKES AN INTEREST GROUP DIFFERENT FROM A POLITICAL PARTY?

Interest groups differ from political parties in several ways. It is important to understand this in order to illustrate strategies interest groups use in seeking to influence decision making. However, as the political author John Kingdom (1991) notes, these differences may not always bear close scrutiny. Unlike political parties, interest groups are not concerned with gaining or keeping legislative power. Instead they are eager to secure government support for their interests in the hope that government policy will be developed accordingly. For example, in furtherance of their interests, trade unions do not put up candidates in general or local elections but may well sponsor individual members of parliament whom they regard as sympathetic and likely to guard or promote union interests. The Society for the Protection of the Unborn Child, on the other hand, has fielded candidates in general elections but they do so in the constituencies of pro-choice members of parliament and their aim is to bring attention to their cause rather than seriously to seek public office.

Unlike political parties who express views on the whole gamut of policies, most interest groups represent a narrow range of interests. For example, groups such as the Alzheimer's Disease Society will be concerned to effect change or influence public policy as it relates to people with Alzheimer's disease, their families, carers and professionals working in the field. They may well articulate views on a range of issues, for example about the funding of clinical research, proposed changes in service delivery or the reduction in carer's allowances. It is unlikely, however, that such a group would try to influence the formulation of industrial policy because it has no direct effect upon the common interest of the group it represents.

Finally, because interest groups aim to influence the development of policy they will seek to inform and collaborate with mainstream political parties whatever their position on the political spectrum. They will try to persuade MPs and all groups that appear to have an effect upon on how policy decisions are made and will seek to exert pressure at various stages of the decision making process. Because policy making is not just confined to central government, interest groups will not direct their attention solely to the politicians at Westminster and the civil servants in Whitehall. Local government and health authorities remain important forums and of course the European Parliament is an increasingly important forum of decision making. Indeed Wallace & Young have identified an increasing number of interest groups setting up offices in Brussels and hiring lobbyists on retainers to ensure that their opinions are heard in the European policy process (Wallace & Young 1996).

TYPOLOGIES OF INTEREST GROUPS

Many attempts have been made to define the essential characteristics of interest group behaviour and in doing so develop a typology of interest groups. It may be of use to look at some of these typologies in order to understand more about the nature of interest groups and how they operate.

Group membership

One obvious way to define interest groups is to look at the membership of the group and the type of interests they articulate. The political theorist Finer (1966) developed a model based on an analysis of whom the group represented. He proposed the following typology:

- the business lobby
- the professional lobby

- the labour lobby

- civic lobbies.

This is clearly a useful way to begin an analysis and provides an initial explanation of interest group behaviour. It is also a model that is easy to apply to those groups that are active in the health policy arena. For example, the *business lobby* clearly encompasses those groups representing commercial interests and would include private health care companies, the pharmaceutical industry and, increasingly, private pension firms. The *professional lobby* by definition would include organizations that represent professional groups such as the Royal College of Nursing, the Community and District Nursing Association and organizations such as the United Kingdom Central Council and the English National Board that have some kind of governing role over a profession. UNISON is an obvious example of an interest group from the *labour lobby*. Finally, Finer identified *civic groups* as a type of interest group. This category may be more difficult to identify but it would include groups that articulate what may be described as altruistic interests, as do charitable groups such as Cancer Relief Macmillan Fund, and MENCAP, which promotes the interests of people with learning disabilities.

Although this typology provides a useful starting point in understanding the activity of interest groups its application is fraught with confusion because of its assumption that organizations can be categorized according to their function and membership. Clearly this is not always so. Attempts to categorize groups in this way may lead to misunderstanding of their function. Indeed an organization may appear to be a classic example of a professional organization but may also exhibit characteristics of a trade union.

The RCN

An obvious example of this split personality is the RCN. Without doubt the RCN is regarded as a professional association, representing and articulating professional issues in public debate. As such, its representatives will be consulted on many issues likely to affect the nursing profession, from changes in the education of nurses to changes in the funding of health and social care services. However, the RCN also represents its members' views on a range of issues that traditionally would be associated with the role of a trade union, for example on pay. The late Trevor Clay (Clay 1987) pointed out that when the RCN adopted the slogan 'The Professional Trade Union for Nurses' it provoked a major wrangle because there were many who thought that the aims of a professional association and those of a trade union were mutually exclusive. The RCN continues to combine both identities.

Temporary and permanent interest groups

The political author Derbyshire (1984) suggests that a more reliable way of classifying interest groups is to define them on the basis of how long they have been established and for how long they are likely to remain in existence. This model acknowledges a distinction between permanent groups representing a long established set of interests and groups that have been established on a temporary basis to represent interests that are transient. In this model, permanent groups are likely to have a national basis. For example the College of Nursing, from which the RCN originates, was established in 1916 and sought to represent all student and registered nurses in the United Kingdom. As such the RCN is clearly an example of a permanent group and can expect to have an active part in the policy process for the foreseeable future.

In this model Derbyshire suggests that temporary interest groups are more likely to articulate local issues. He suggests that such groups are likely to be formed for a short term and are likely to disappear once the issue has been resolved. The Snowdrop appeal was established in 1996 in Dunblane to campaign for changes in the gun laws. The group achieved partial success under a Conservative government but persuaded the opposition Labour Party to support its call for a total ban on the private ownership of handguns. Following the election of a new Labour government in May 1997 and an announcement of changes to the Firearms Amendment Bill the Snowdrop appeal was wound up.

This model may help to explain why it is that some interest groups which appear to have a high visibility at one moment may suddenly disappear from view. However, this model does not explain why some groups which appear to have some measure of permanence in terms of their structure and membership seem not to have success in influencing the formulation of policy. For example, the Society for the Protection of the Unborn Child has been in existence for many years and has a national membership. Nevertheless, although it is very vocal and enjoys the backing of some MPs its influence on abortion policy has to date been limited.

Insider/outsider groups

A more useful way of defining interest groups which begins to address some of the criticisms that I have identified has been called the insider/outsider model. This model postulates that interest groups can be differentiated in terms of their relationship to the policy making process and begins to explain why some groups appear to have more success than others in influencing government policy. The greater the involvement a group has with government suggests the degree to which it is 'inside the decision making process'. Kingdom (1991) suggests that the factors that determine insider status include: whether the group is held in high public esteem; whether or not it espouses an ideology or cause that is fairly close to that prevailing in current political parties; whether its core values reflect mainstream social values; and, finally, whether it can command economic or political leverage.

Using this model, an interest group can be identified as an insider group if it actively takes part in the formulation of policy, for example if a representative of the group is asked to be an expert witness before a parliamentary select committee. The British Medical Association (BMA) is a good example of an insider group. The BMA represents a group of professionals that is held in high public esteem, it espouses interests that reflect mainstream social values and it appears to command considerable political leverage. Clearly a government proposing to make changes to the way health care is provided would ensure that representatives of this group were consulted and that their views informed the decisions made. In contrast to insider groups, outsider groups are not actively involved in policy formation, either by design or consequence. They are not seen as obvious members of the policy making process.

One of the appeals of this typology of interest groups is that it recognizes the dynamic nature of a modern democracy as a developing entity rather than a static formal process with predetermined actors. It begins to allow us to understand why some groups appear to be more involved with the policy process at a given time. For example, trade unions representing health care workers have, historically, played a more central role in the formulation of health policy under

Labour governments because of their shared vision of the NHS. However, during the 1990s health reforms presided over by a Conservative government, the unions were marginalized because of their opposition to the reforms.

Types of insider group

The insider/outsider typology is further developed by Maloney et al (1994) who suggest that insider groups can be divided into: core insider groups, specialist insider groups, and peripheral insider groups.

Core insider groups. In applying this model to the health service, core insiders will be those groups which are believed to have an important contribution to make on a host of issues and as such are frequently consulted. The Royal College of Nursing is an example of a core insider group. Representatives of this organization are regularly asked to contribute their views on a range of subjects from the development of the primary care White Paper (Butler 1997) through to the development of policy that addresses the needs of people with HIV.

Specialist insider groups. Specialist insider groups are defined, as the name suggests, as groups who have specialist knowledge and will be consulted periodically on issues that relate to that specific area of knowledge. For example, Cancer Relief will be asked to submit views on a range of issues that relate to cancer, from the development of screening programmes to the formulation of healthy eating programmes, but they are unlikely to be consulted over proposals to change the national pay structures of nurses.

Peripheral insider groups. Peripheral groups will also be acknowledged to have access to specialist knowledge but their knowledge relates to an even smaller area of policy. Maloney suggests that consultation with these groups will often be cosmetic, in other words the importance of consulting them will have more to do with name checking the organization than actually listening to them in any detail. Examples of this group may be harder to identify simply because no one would want to admit such cosmetic and limited involvement. However, one could argue that, historically, groups representing the views of alternative therapists, such as osteopaths, would once have been treated as peripheral insider groups although their position has undergone change towards greater acceptance of their specialist knowledge, as the 1993 Osteopaths Act and the subsequent establishment of the first General Osteopathic Council in 1996 testifies: yet another manifestation of dynamism.

Types of outsider group

Maloney et al (1994) posit that outsider groups can be split into two camps: outsider group by ideology and outsider group by choice. The outsider group by ideology refers to groups whose aims are unlikely to be achieved in the traditional policy making process. The interests they espouse are more likely to necessitate structural changes to society rather than minor policy changes. The King's Cross Women's Centre have long campaigned for women's work within the home to be financially rewarded in recognition of its contribution to the national economy. This demand is unlikely to be fully achieved without a major reshaping of public finance; clearly this represents a radical change in philosophy and as a consequence the group remains outside the policy making community. The outsider group by choice refers to groups that do not actively seek to have a close relationship with policy making despite their presence in the wider field. The activity of some anarchist networks in the anti-road movement is an example of this second group. Although they are very active in the campaign they appear not to want a close relationship with the formal political system, leaving this role to more established interest groups, for example the Society for the Protection of Rural Britain, within the movement.

Clearly, at the heart of the insider/outsider model is the notion that interest groups that pursue a cause that in reality is close to what the formal actors view as possible policy will be most likely to be given an insider position, of whatever type.

HOW DO INTEREST GROUPS OPERATE?

I have demonstrated that interest groups exist to represent the views of a particular group within society. But whom do they seek to influence and what strategies do they adopt to achieve this?

I have already suggested that the flow of benefits between interest groups and the formal actors involved in making decisions is a two-way process. Not only do interest groups seek to influence the making of policy but the formal actors often recognize the merit of involving them because they may possess expert knowledge which other parties lack and which may have bearing on decisions. The formal actors will seek to tap into this unique knowledge or experience in order to strengthen the decision making process.

Influencing political parties

Let us consider the process of how an interest group will seek to exert its influence proactively over decision making. In a mature Western democracy there are many ways of doing this. Firstly, let us consider how to persuade political parties. One of the most obvious strategies has been to sponsor, or in some way financially support, the work of an individual member of parliament (MP). For example, trade unions have historically sponsored individual MPs in the hope that they will present the union's views when policy is being discussed. The deputy leader of the Labour Party, John Prescott, is sponsored by the Transport and General Workers Union (TGWU) and has long articulated the interests of TGWU members in transport debates within Parliament.

Another way to ensure that a particular issue is heard is for a representative of an interest group to become either a formal or informal adviser to one of the major parties. For example, in 1992, the chair of the Patients' Association helped to write the Conservative Party health manifesto and the president of the Community and District Nursing Association, Ann Keen, has in the past been Labour's nursing adviser (Butler 1997). In 1997 Ann Keen was elected as an MP with a personal mandate to ensure that nursing had a voice in Parliament.

Parliamentary lobbyists

The larger interest groups may well employ lobbyists whose job it will be to develop and maintain working links with individual MPs and the political parties to ensure that the views of the group are represented. For example, many of the major charities employ parliamentary officers whose job it is to keep the organization up to date with what is going on at Westminster as well as to develop a relationship with MPs or party officials so that they can feed their views into policy debates. The RCN employs a parliamentary and media team whose job it is to provide the organization with an authoritative and effective voice in Parliament as well as in the media. This tactic is also used by interest groups representing commercial interests who commonly employ the services of a professional lobbyist firm. Increasingly, this last type of representation is being called into question because of growing unease about its propriety, the so-called 'cash for questions' scenario.

Smaller interest groups with fewer financial resources often rely on their own members to lobby politicians. For example, they ask members to take part in letter writing campaigns to their own MPs in the hope that an MP deluged with letters about the closure of a local hospital will either raise the matter in the House of Commons or intervene at local level. Other interest groups may look for a sympathetic partner financially and administratively to support a campaign. Breast cancer groups and anti-domestic violence groups have worked with the Body Shop to raise awareness of these issues and have run postcard campaigns from their shops.

Influencing civil servants

Interest groups recognize that another important set of actors in the policy making process are the non-elected government officers because it is at the departmental level that policy will be formulated. Many civil servants will have a longer career within a department than the relevant minister, who may at any time move departments in a cabinet reshuffle. So, some interest groups will develop a working relationship with key civil servants who hold a particular policy portfolio and will regularly send them briefings to ensure that their views remain on the agenda.

Influencing the media

Interest groups will also seek to influence people outside the formal political arenas, people whom they believe have access to, or indeed may have influence over decision taking. For example, interest groups may seek to harness the power of the media to reach a wider audience. An interest group may well tip off a newspaper about a demonstration in anticipation that they will receive media coverage and in so doing inform the general public and enlist their support. A rally by the Save Barts Hospital group, held outside the Conservative Party Headquarters during the 1997 election campaign, was clearly an attempt to publicize the group's cause through the media. Organizations campaigning to raise awareness about particular health issues have increasingly turned to television as a way of highlighting issues, either in the form of a documentary or as a story line in a prime-time soap opera. HIV, breast cancer and schizophrenia have all featured in major television story lines and representatives from particular interest groups have sometimes been involved in advising producers of programmes about how best a subject might be presented (Stokes 1997).

Providing expert knowledge

I discussed earlier how the relationship between interest groups and policy makers is a two-way affair. Not only do interest groups actively seek ways of influencing policy making, but also those who make decisions seek out the views of interest groups. The nature of British democracy is such that MPs and civil servants do not have specific expert knowledge over the whole policy range and will therefore identify expertise in a variety of settings, including academia and interest groups. As experts are identified, they may be informally consulted on a particular matter or they may formally be called to give evidence to a select committee. The Conservative government sought advice from some of the most influential interest groups before it began to formulate the 1990 NHS and Community Care Act. Groups are consulted not only because they have expert knowledge but also because it is thought better to have them on board during discussions than have them agitating and possibly even undermining the development of policy from outside. Clearly interest groups are an important resource to government, offering expert advice and information on particular issues at little expense to government.

WHY DO INTEREST GROUPS CHOOSE A PARTICULAR STRATEGY?

The chosen strategy by which an interest group will advance its cause will vary greatly to suit not only the group's particular aims at the time but also to accommodate their own perception of their current relationship with government. For example, interest groups which appear to occupy what we have called an outsider position may choose openly to confront government by mobilizing public support for their views if they feel it unlikely that the government of the day will listen sympathetically. Recent campaigns protesting against closure of inner city hospitals have actively sought to mobilize public opinion through public meetings, demonstrations and letter-writing campaigns. In doing so they clearly hoped that subsequent pressure on government ministers would prove irresistible.

So far in this chapter I have tried to demonstrate that the British political system is not just the preserve of formal political parties and that an individual's ability to take part in politics is not restricted to voting in a general election every 5 years. Many groups articulating a variety of different interests seek to influence the political process in the hope that their views will positively affect the formulation of policy. Crudely, these interest groups seek to influence policy making either by working with political parties, for example by participating in relevant committees, or advising political parties, or seeking to lobby politicians from outside the system. It is widely acknowledged that the existence of interest groups has become an important feature of postwar British politics (Kingdom 1991). But how can we explain this phenomenon? How have interest groups become so important in the political system?

PLURALISM

The dominant explanation of the increasing activity of interest groups has been that of pluralism. A pluralist political system is usually described as one in which there is no dominant political, ideological or cultural group. Pluralists postulate that society, and therefore the political process, is open and, as an expression of that openness, all individuals have the same access to the decision making process. Within the pluralist model, government is thought to be neutral. Policy is formed by ministers listening to and arbitrating between the views of different groups and individual actors in what some commentators have suggested is almost a policy bazaar. Dearlove, for example, suggests that pluralists view the political process as an idealized economic marketplace of free and fair competition where all interest groups have the same opportunity to shape public policy (Dearlove & Saunders 1991).

Pluralists would argue that an individual's ability to participate in the political process is not limited simply to voting in the general election. This would be seen as a very limited notion of democracy. In contrast, they would argue that the structure of our political system offers greater opportunities to affect policy making, for example by lobbying government ministers or by taking part in parliamentary select committees. Pluralists maintain that all individuals can affect the workings of the political system but they will have a greater chance of influencing policy if they band together with other like-minded people in order to promote their ideas within government. Indeed the existence of such groups is thought to strengthen the democratic credentials of a society. In other words, a pluralist society becomes defined by the existence of a multiplicity of interest groups articulating a variety of concerns within the policy making forum.

In this model, interest groups exist almost as an expression of the openness of the democratic political system. The activity of interest groups is therefore thought to support the democratic process because it affords individuals greater opportunities to affect what policies are made. The process of bartering between groups is also thought to increase the likelihood of formulating policy by consensus. This is believed to be so because the model ensures, at least theoretically, that a wide range of views is heard by government ministers; it thus ensures that groups feel that they have participated in the process and therefore are more likely to accept the outcome.

Pluralists argue that within the political system no dominant interest group exists. They suggest that all groups are equal and that no hierarchy exists between the groups. There is a balance of power between groups because they have equal access to influencing policy. Because, pluralists maintain, all interests groups have free access to decision making, politics, being fluid, can change overnight, and the policy process is best characterized as one involving negotiation and bargaining.

Is the pluralist interpretation adequate?

Does the pluralist interpretation adequately explain this aspect of the British political system and the role of interest groups? Is it realistic to suggest that government is neutral and that all interest groups exert the same degree of influence over the policy making process? Let us look at these questions more closely.

Neutrality

It would be difficult to deny that political parties, whether in government or opposition, have established theoretical positions which they seek to pursue. All governments appear to have views on what type of policies should be developed, based on a particular theoretical position, and therefore have inherent bias. In an analysis of how decisions are made within the health policy field, Butler & Vaile (1984) argue that those involved in policy formation have vested interests to preserve and that sometimes they are keener to pursue these interests than they are in developing policy that reflects the views of competing groups. Indeed, the Conservative governments of 1979–1997 maintained an explicit commitment to rolling back the welfare state which was based on a theoretical position of the reassertion of market principles to all areas of the public sector (Johnson 1991).

They did so against a backdrop of criticism and opposition from a variety of sources.

Equality

Secondly, it would appear simplistic to suggest that all interest groups have equal power to effect changes. Clearly some groups have more influence over policy making than others do. Under the pluralist model one would expect groups that represent the greatest number of people to have the greatest influence in the policy making process, maintaining what Kingdom has called the democratic principle of majoritarianism. However, this is clearly not so. Some groups have a degree of influence far out of proportion to the size of their membership. For example, if majoritarianism held, then one would expect the RCN, which represents the largest proportion of health care professionals working in the NHS, to have as much influence, if not more, than the BMA. Few would agree that it does, except on rare occasions.

What determines influence?

The degree of influence that an interest group wields changes over time and is dependent on many factors, not just the political hue of the government of the day. Some interest groups clearly have greater influence and are more likely than others to be consulted because of perceived notions of power. It might be that they are thought to wield significant economic leverage which may need to be harnessed to the cause or that they have some professional leverage which will be important in securing changes to policy. Clearly the NHS was established by ensuring that the medical profession was brought on board rather than their being in total opposition to the proposal.

The success of a particular interest group is often determined by its ability to play the game, for example, to have the financial resources necessary to lobby government both formally and informally or to have the knowledge, experience and confidence to take part in the process. Arguably this system tends to perpetuate the marginalization of interest groups that represent people who are already marginalized in society. Organizations representing issues of specific concern to black people or the homeless may lack the financial resources to engage the political system. Similarly, groups representing young people may lack the experience necessary to coordinate an effective lobbying programme. A weakness shows up when groups continue to be ignored because government ministers, MPs and civil servants feel no compulsion to listen to their views and are thus able to ignore them. Without doubt this is the fate of some small interest groups that deserve a hearing. It is only slightly less discouraging when consultation is cosmetic and carries no weight.

Smaller groups representing the interests of marginalized groups often struggle to be heard, even though they raise legitimate concerns. The system of government in Britain is not in reality able to deal with all the interest groups that exist. Preferences are formed that may reflect political, economic or cultural views. For example, ministers reviewing mental health services may well prioritize the professional views of psychiatrists and community psychiatric nurses over the lay wishes of survivor networks. Not all groups share the same access or influence over government. As already stated, some groups will be consulted in a cosmetic fashion rather than in any meaningful sense and others may simply be ignored.

Some groups, however, that have historically been marginalized by the policy making community have nevertheless been able to develop a measure of influence when the issues that they raise become more important to a majority of the population. Groups such as the Terrence Higgins Trust and the Lighthouse have worked hard at raising awareness about the implications that HIV raises for mainstream health policy and have become effective in lobbying for changes in health promotion and in the way clinical research is funded. Similarly, issues that have in the past been ignored may be treated with greater respect by a new government, for example the new Labour government has joined forces with the mental health charity Mind to tackle concerns over the delivery of mental health services to black people (McMillan 1997).

CORPORATISM

The pluralist explanation of interest group activity is flawed because it fails adequately to explain how some groups appear to have more success in influencing policy than others, and also because it is based on an unsubstantiated view of government as a neutral arbitrator. With these criticisms in mind, some commentators have used a corporatist analysis to explain why some interest groups appear more successful than others.

As a theoretical explanation of interest group activity, corporatism rests on an assumption that government is not neutral and that it works in close cooperation with major interest groups within society to develop policy in line with its own beliefs. However, the basic assumption is that those interest groups working closely with government do so in a collective manner, working with each other rather than against each other. In other words, interest groups are brought into the political process and incorporated as active participants rather than as willing subordinates (Middlemas 1979).

Commentators on the British political system (Middlemas 1979, Crouch 1982) point to the tripartite relationship between government, business and labour that characterized industrial relations in the 1960s and early 1970s as evidence to support the idea of corporatism. Clearly the assumption is that interest groups will work with government so long as there is some shared notion of a common vision. Once that vision is removed the groups will no longer work in close cooperation with government. With respect to the incorporation of trade unions, it is thought that this was based on a shared ideal of full employment. However, once the government changed and this ideal dropped from its political consciousness, the trade union movement was no longer seen as an important partner.

With the corporatist explanation in mind one can see evidence of some interest groups having been integrated into the health policy making process at the expense of other groups. For example the RCN clearly enjoyed a closer relationship with the Conservative government of 1979–1997 than many other interest groups representing health professionals. Indeed, even the BMA, which historically enjoys a close relationship with government, had for a time a more adversarial relationship with government ministers and frequently criticized government reforms of the NHS. In their analysis of British political life from Callaghan to Thatcher, Derbyshire & Derbyshire (1990) point out that after the publication of the 1989 White Paper *Working for patients*, the BMA ran an advertising campaign against the government's reforms and that some critics went as far as forming an NHS supporters party which put forward candidates in parliamentary by-elections (Derbyshire & Derbyshire 1990). At the same time, those groups representing the views of doctors who supported the NHS reforms appeared to have had a much closer relationship with health ministers (Butler

1997). In essence, those groups which are incorporated into the political system will continue to work with government so long as they enjoy a pay-off. Once this is removed the relationship is likely to break down.

The corporatist model recognizes that the involvement of interest groups is a two-way process. Interest groups can influence the formation of policy and government can, in exchange, influence the way interest groups behave and can force them to alter their demands, or behave in a way that is thought to be more appropriate. However, it may be impossible to explain the behaviour of all interest groups with reference to one theoretical model. In reality, groups are established, influence the formation of policy, or not, in multifarious ways, being themselves subject to a host of factors, external and internal. The ability of an individual interest group to influence policy making will alter over time to reflect changes in government, changes in party policy, shifting ministerial loyalties and the mood of the country. Any analysis of their behaviour needs to reflect this dynamic.

CONCLUSION

The chapter began with an exploration of the nature of interest groups and their role within the policy making process. Several typologies of interest groups were identified and critiques advanced in order that the reader might begin to develop the tools necessary to examine the nature of individual groups; for example, to understand why some groups appear to have a permanent existence whilst others may only exist for a matter of months or years.

We then went on to look at the different strategies that groups might use to promote their views and we contem-

plated the relationship between interest groups and the policy making process. Finally, we began to consider some of
the theoretical explanations of their development within the
British political system. In the process, we hope to have
prompted readers to reflect upon their own relationship
with the political process and also to consider the professional organizations, trade unions and other groups to
which they may belong and which may function as interest
groups.

Interest groups would seem to have become an integral part
of the political process. They improve governance by providing a source of current expert knowledge which government ministers and civil servants can hardly be expected to
possess. They can also be established quickly in response to
a particular incident (Snowdrop/Dunblane) and can
demonstrate current concerns within society. In that sense
their existence provides a flexibility that the formal policy
making process may fail to allow. Most importantly they
can act as intermediary groups between the people and government, a channel for communication of ideas. Many
groups that represent the views of patients and carers (e.g.
MIND) already establish a framework that enables individuals to articulate their position and ensure that their views
are heard.

Not only do interest groups provide a means by which individuals can participate at one remove in the activities of
government, but they are structured channels for communication, an instant sounding board against which government can test ideas. Larger, well established interest groups
with permanent parliamentary officers can also act as
watch-dogs over public policy in its formation, ensuring
that relevant organizations are aware of proposed legislation. Parliamentary officers at the RCN will no doubt try to
inform the widest possible audience about issues that they

think are of concern not only to their members but also to the relevant special interest groups, patient groups and, possibly, other trade unions.

The existence of interest groups can also weaken democracy in that their marginal existence might encourage governments to sideline particular issues. Rather than bringing issues of concern to the heart of the political consciousness they can be used as token experts, to be kept at arm's length but brought in at a particularly sensitive moment. Within the health policy arena we have already identified a number of groups that in the past have been sidelined but currently appear to be more involved in policy formation, for example groups representing alternative therapists and specific patient groups. The 1990s move towards greater and more visible consultation may have ensured that a greater number of interest groups have been brought into the policy formation process, but we must ask whether they have really played an active role.

A caution – interest groups in the health service, as elsewhere, often deal with specific special interests and so balance must be kept between them. Some groups are better at voicing their views than others, so it is important to ensure also that professional views are considered in the light of patients' opinions.

In short, involvement of interest groups is a means by which functions of government and wider expertise are brought together by non-governmental agency. Clearly, participation in interest groups is a significant way of raising important issues. The Association of Radical Midwives has long campaigned to change the way in which midwifery services are provided in Britain and their report, *The vision* (Association of Radical Midwives 1986), was influential in the development of the *Changing childbirth*

(Department of Health 1993) report. These opportunities to influence policy making must be grasped. Often it is those who are closest to an issue, either because they are professionals working in the service or because they are recipients of the service, who have the necessary knowledge and motivation to promote change.

■ QUESTIONS FOR DISCUSSION

- What is the relationship between interest groups and the policy making process?
- What strategies might interest groups use to influence the political process?
- Has the RCN's dual role, as a professional association and a trade union, had an impact on its effectiveness in promoting the interests of nurses and nursing?
- How might nurses increase their effectiveness in lobbying on behalf of their patients/clients?

FURTHER READING

Kingdom J 1991 Government and politics in Britain. Polity Press, Cambridge

An interesting and lively introduction to the political process in Britain. The author uses imaginative sources to illustrate the points under discussion.

Maloney W A, Jordan G, McLaughlin A 1994 Interest groups and public policy: the insider/outsider model revisited. Journal of Public Policy 14(1):17–38

A key academic text in the study of the interest group behaviour.

Clay T 1987 Nurses, power and politics. Heinemann, London

A classic which explores the relationship between nursing, nurses and the political process.

Ham C 1992 Health policy in Britain: the politics and organisation of the National Health Service. Macmillan, London

A comprehensive assessment of the development of the NHS. The book provides many examples of how interest groups have influenced the policy making process.

REFERENCES

Association of Radical Midwives 1986 The vision – proposals for the future of the maternity services. ARM, Ormskirk

Butler J, Vaile S 1984 Health and health services: an introduction to health care in Britain. Routledge and Kegan Paul, London

Butler P 1997 Heard but not seen. Health Service Journal 107(5544):15

Clay T 1987 Nurses, power and politics. Heinemann, London

Crouch C 1982 The politics of industrial relations. Fontana, Suffolk

Dearlove J, Saunders P 1991 Introduction to British politics, 2nd edn. Polity Press, Cambridge

Derbyshire J D 1984 An introduction to public administration, 2nd edn. McGraw-Hill, London

Derbyshire J D, Derbyshire I 1990 Politics in Britain: from Callaghan to Thatcher. Chambers, Edinburgh

Department of Health 1993 Changing childbirth. Report of the Expert Maternity Group. HMSO, London

Finer S 1966 Anonymous empire. Pall Mall Press, London

Johnson N 1991 The break-up of consensus: competitive politics in a declining economy. In: Loney M, Bocock R, Clarke J, Cochrane A, Gaham P, Wilson M (eds) The state or the market: politics and welfare in contemporary Britain. Sage, London, ch 12, p 214

Kingdom J 1991 Government and politics in Britain. Polity Press, Cambridge

McMillan I 1997 Changing minds. Nursing Standard 11(52):14

Maloney W A, Jordan G, McLaughlin A 1994 Interest groups and public policy: the insider/outsider model revisited. Journal of Public Policy 14(1):17–38

Masterson A 1994 Making and implementing social policy. In: Gough P, Maslin-Prothero S, Masterson A (eds) Nursing and social policy. Butterworth-Heinemann, Oxford, ch 2, p 32

Middlemas K 1979 Politics in industrial society. Deutsch, London

Stokes R 1997 A guy named Joe. Nursing Standard 11(39):17

Wallace H, Young A R 1996 The single market approach to policy. In: Wallace H, Wallace W (eds) Policy making in the European Union. Oxford University Press, Oxford, ch 5, p 125

The role of local government

Linda East

INTRODUCTION

The purpose of this chapter is to introduce the reader to the role of local government in British politics and to identify the interfaces between local government, health and nursing. Like nursing, local government does not always enjoy a high public profile. In 1992 the Royal College of Nursing (RCN) suggested that 'so much of what nurses do is invisible. Good nursing care is often demonstrated by the fact that you can't see it' (RCN 1992, p. 1). Similar claims have been made for local government:

At the heart of council operations are those 'invisible' services on which civilised life depends, from street lighting to parks maintenance. They are invisible because, for most people, they have long entered the arena of things-taken-for-granted, things noticed only when they are suddenly not there – when the pavement is up, when the bins are not emptied, when the street is dark. (Walker 1996, p. 10)

The number of voters who turn out for local elections is, on average, only half the number of those who vote in national elections. When it is possible to travel round the world just by switching on the television it is, perhaps, not surprising that people do not get too excited at the prospect of voting in the occupants of their town halls. However, the adage 'think globally, act locally' is instructive. Local services do matter, and local government plays a major role in promoting and maintaining health. To be healthy, people need a voice in decision making and a sense of control over the forces which shape their lives. Healthy communities need jobs, houses, schools, shops, roads and parks. Local authorities are responsible not only for the direct provision of services but also for creating a climate in which individuals and communities can prosper.

My aim is to provide readers of this chapter with a sense of how these activities fit together and the ways in which nurses can access and exploit local authority services for the benefit of themselves and their clients. To this end, the rest of the chapter will consider four crucial areas. First, I will endeavour to address the question 'what exactly is local government?' Like all complex institutions, it is easy to get bogged down in the detail and lose a sense of the larger picture. However, I want readers to see that they are not dealing with an impenetrable monolith but with an organization they have the potential to influence. For nurses and others whose life's work is promoting health and alleviating sickness, the starting point must be our own role as citizens and active members of the society in which we live. I will then move on to consider two broad areas of local authority activity which are of great relevance to nurses and health workers, namely public health and the personal social services. I will conclude by highlighting some of the areas in which health services and local authorities might work together to promote health and the ways in which nurses might engage with the political processes of local government.

WHAT IS LOCAL GOVERNMENT?

In his excellent introductory text, *Local government today*, Chandler (1996) states that 'local government is a unique and valuable institution' (p. 1). He defines the remit of local government as follows:

> *In Britain, local government refers to the authorities and*
> *dependent agencies that are established, according to*
> *legislation and statute, under the direction of a locally elected*
> *council to provide services for their localities and to represent*
> *their interests (Chandler 1996, p. 1).*

Not all authors would accept that local government is restricted only to the authorities that work under the direction of a locally elected council. Stoker (1991), for example, argues that local government encompasses both elected and non-elected authorities. He points out that organizations such as health authorities and police authorities have an important role in developing and implementing locality-specific policies in partnership with local councils.

Similarly, local businesses, voluntary and campaigning

groups contribute their own unique perspective to the leadership of towns and cities. However, the idea that local government is elected is a recurrent theme in many definitions (Cole & Boyne 1995). If we also accept that local government exercises jurisdiction over a smaller area than national government, has powers of taxation, and has discretion over service provision we arrive at a working definition of local government adequate for the purposes of this chapter.

I should, perhaps, at this point offer the reader some explanation as to why I am writing this chapter and my qualifications for so doing. Like many nurses who completed their training in London in the 1980s, I am something of a political animal and have held a long-standing membership of the Labour Party (I make this clear so the reader can weigh up the influence of party politics in my arguments for local government). In 1995 I was selected by my local Labour Party to stand for election as a City of Nottingham councillor. I was duly elected, and have since spent much of my spare time engaged in the various activities which being a councillor entails (summarized in Fig. 5.1). I take personal experience as my starting point because I believe the British system of government, both locally and nationally, can seem very remote and difficult to understand. How do people become councillors or members of parliament? What are their responsibilities and how are they called to account? It is just these questions I will now seek to address.

As Chapter 3 will have made clear, the starting point for most politicians, local and national, is membership of one of the major political parties. It is, of course, possible to stand for election as an independent candidate. The election of journalist Martin Bell as member of parliament for Tatton in 1997 demonstrates that people are willing to vote for an independent candidate with a clear message and a high

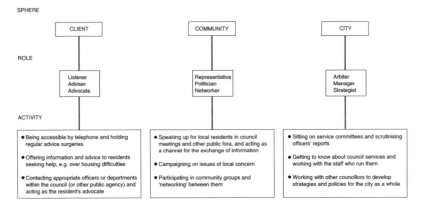

Fig. 5.1 The city councillor's role and sphere of activities.

profile. However, for most would-be independent politicians the chances of getting elected are slim at the level of a parliamentary constituency and still fairly remote at the level of the electoral ward which councillors represent. In the case of candidates standing on a party slate, electors should have a reasonable idea of what the parties stand for and the policies they will seek to implement in office. In the case of independent candidates, on the other hand, the electorate is likely to require a more personal knowledge of their potential representative in order to establish what they stand for. So, for most councillors, the route into local government is via selection as a candidate by the local branch of their political party and subsequent election at the polls. Periods of office are generally 3 years, with many authorities electing a third of their councillors on an annual basis, ensuring continuity and offering electors a more frequent opportunity to vote. Once in office, councillors are ultimately responsible and accountable to the electorate for the services their authority delivers. Of course, professional officers with extensive training and expertise support them. However, officers are essentially civil servants who are expected to take their strategic direction from the policies laid out in the majority party's manifesto.

As a result of the local selection and election processes outlined above, local government in the UK is nearly always run along party lines. The majority party takes control of the council, which means it elects the leader, deputy leader and the chairs of committees. However, it should be noted that there is, at present, no equivalent to the Cabinet in national government at the local level. All councillors take decisions and there is no executive tier within local councils. There is continual debate over extending efficiency and accountability in local government and proposals for directly elected mayors of towns and cities are gaining favour (Wilson & Game 1994). Nothing in local government stands still for long, as the following paragraphs outlining the historical development of local government in the UK will show.

THE HISTORICAL DEVELOPMENT OF LOCAL GOVERNMENT IN THE UK

Parishes

Britain is a country where church and state have been closely intertwined in shaping our history. In medieval times through to the 19th century, the parish church was the locus for local debate and decision making. Parishes were charged with the responsibility of supporting the infirm through the mechanisms of the Elizabethan Poor Law of 1601, which endowed an individual's parish of origin with an enduring significance as the place of last resort should personal misfortune strike. The citizens appointed to office within the parish were invariably the local gentry and landowners, aided by the local parson who was often a dignitary in his own right.

Counties

If the parishes were fora for local decision making, the other arm of historical local government was very much concerned with maintaining central government's control of the shires. The historical role of the British county was to ensure the maintenance of law and order through the actions of the sheriff, lord lieutenant and justices of the peace. The county sheriffs and lord lieutenants, in particular, were local nobility who often held seats in Parliament. They were direct deputies for the monarch and had the power to enforce the law of the land. Vestiges of this power can be seen today, for it is the county sheriff who confronts 'eco-warriors' protesting against the building of new roads and runways, and who is responsible for overseeing the eviction of such protesters from their tree tops and tunnels. In history, too, the parishes and counties were often in conflict and parishes were subject to close observation and supervision by the justices of the peace (Chandler 1996).

Town councils

The tradition of independent town councils developed alongside the system of parishes and counties. It was possible for towns to secure independence following the granting of a Royal Charter, usually as a reward for some service to the Crown. Here too, however, a self-perpetuating élite rather than a democratically elected body of councillors exercised government, with local businessmen and landowners dominating. It was not until the pressures of rapid urbanization and industrialization began to bite in the 18th and 19th centuries that the wheels of reform were set in motion. By this time the parishes were not an effectual unit of government as they were unable to support the numbers of impoverished people displaced as a consequence of increasing labour mobility. The Poor Law Amendment Act of 1834 effectively abolished the operational role of the parish in local government by making much larger unions of parishes responsible for the administration of Poor Law Relief.

Reform

About the same time, the growth of business entrepreneurship highlighted the ineffectual role of the non-elected town councils and the pressures for reform mounted. The Municipal Corporations Act of 1835, building on the Electoral Reform Act of 1832, allowed larger cities to become boroughs governed by representative councils and set out the rules for the foundation of new municipalities. These changes paved the way for locally elected town, city and county councils and the modern system of local government was born.

THE STRUCTURE AND FUNCTIONS OF LOCAL AUTHORITIES IN THE UK

However, debate as to the correct size and composition of local authorities has never really ceased. Numerous reorganizations throughout the 20th century have highlighted that there is no consensus over the ultimate remit for local government in the UK. Demands to remould the structures created in the late 19th century into yet larger units appeared soon after the First World War. Cities had grown into urban conurbations governed by several independent local authorities. The reformers argued that this made it difficult to plan for cities as a whole because so many independent councils had to agree, and because the size of many units was too small to employ economies of scale or to serve special needs (Chandler 1996).

Perhaps the apotheosis of such arguments was reached in the London Government Act of 1963, which abolished the county councils of London and Middlesex to create the Greater London Council (GLC). The purpose of the GLC was to plan and deliver services for London as whole, taking on a powerful strategic and coordinating role. The same Act reduced the number of lower tier authorities from over 100 to just 32 London boroughs, again in acknowledgement of arguments for efficiency of scale in service delivery. However, as any Londoners reading this chapter will know, the reign of the GLC was relatively short-lived. Local elections often produce an administration of the opposing political hue to the central government of the time, partly reflecting the electorate's registering of a 'protest vote' and, perhaps, also registering the commitment of British voters to political pluralism. However, the open opposition of the Labour-controlled GLC to the national Conservative administrations of the 1980s became too much for central government to take and, amid widespread protest, the Greater London Council was abolished in 1986. It has been argued that this leaves a vacuum in the government of our capital city and the debate as to the appropriate form and function of the local authority in London is far from over. The Labour government elected in 1997 has promised to reinstate some form of capital-wide local government as part of a 'new deal for London', though the precise structure and functions of the proposed authority are not clear at the time of writing (Labour Party 1997).

New thinking on the appropriate size of local authorities for efficient and cost-effective service delivery has also resulted in changes in other parts of the country. Recent reorganizations in England have followed the recommendations of the Local Government Commission set up in the early 1990s to examine local authority boundaries. The Local Government Commission favoured granting unitary status to as many councils as possible on the grounds that a single-tier system would reduce running costs and bureaucracy, improve coordination of services and increase accountability to the local electorate (Byrne 1994). The unitary system makes a single local authority responsible for all the services within its boundaries, thus abolishing the old two-tier system, which divided responsibilities between district and county councils. To take Nottinghamshire as an example, the impact of these changes on the organization of local government is profound. Between 1974 and 1998, Nottinghamshire County Council was responsible for the strategic and operational management of large-scale services across the county, including education, social services and transport. However, the Local Government Commission recommended that the City of Nottingham be granted unitary status, which means that those services provided by the county council within its boundaries will be transferred to the city council. Thus, the residents of Nottingham City will receive the services administered by local government from a single, unitary authority – although the city boundaries are somewhat arbitrary and exclude many people who would define themselves as city residents. Nottinghamshire County Council, on the other hand, will continue to deliver its current raft of services to the remaining two-thirds of the residents of Nottinghamshire. The district authorities outside the City of Nottingham will also continue to deliver the services for which they are responsible, including housing, refuse collection and leisure services. This will no doubt cause some confusion to health workers, who operate on completely different boundaries again. For example, purchasing community care services for the area covered by Nottingham Health Authority currently involves negotiations with no less than six different local authorities. In many parts of the country, health and local authority boundaries bear little relationship to each other.

The new single-tier urban authorities are, of course, emerging throughout the country and not just in Nottinghamshire. Some of the counties created by the local government reorganizations of the 1970s (for example Avon and Cleveland) have been written out of the new map of local government, with cities such as Bristol gaining the status of unitary authorities. The reorganization of local government in Scotland and Wales, on the other hand, meant unitary authorities came into being much earlier. In Wales, many of the smaller districts were abolished or amalgamated so that authorities which were county councils prior to 1974 took on the responsibilities of the smaller district authorities. In Scotland, on the other hand, the larger regions were abolished and their powers were transferred to the districts to create the Scottish unitary authorities (Chandler 1996). It remains to be seen whether the widespread adoption of the unitary model will result in the increased local efficiency and accountability that supporters predict. However, it is unlikely that the pressures for the continual reshaping and refining of local government boundaries and functions will end here. Proposals for Scottish and Welsh devolution and for a new tier of regional government may well alter the maps once more.

THE CHANGING ROLE OF LOCAL GOVERNMENT

It should be clear from the above paragraphs that many of the forces which shape local government in the UK reflect the search for the ideal size and structure of a local authority which will deliver services efficiently and effectively. However, the form which local government takes at any given time is also responsive to the political ideologies held by national governments. Many writers in this field characterize the 1980s as a time when local and central governments were frequently in conflict, with the latter attempting to redefine the remit and responsibilities of the former. It should be noted that local councils have no special constitutional position which protects their status and role within the UK system of government. Local government is subject to the sovereign will of Parliament, in particular the law of *ultra vires*, which holds local authorities can only do that which is permitted to them by statute law (Hill 1994).

In a paper entitled 'Is there a future for local government?' Cochrane (1992) argues that it is disingenuous to suggest that central government is the villain in the war of attrition against local government. It was widely acknowledged by all political parties in the 1980s that the calibre of local government officers and councillors could be improved upon, and that private sector management models had something to offer local bureaucracies. Our 20th-century local government systems developed as part of the welfare state, and are subject both to economic retrenchment and to changing beliefs among policy makers as to the fundamental beliefs upon which social policies are based (Le Grand 1997). In the health service, we have seen the emergence of quasi-markets whereby hospitals have become independent provider trusts in competition for contracts with the commissioning health authorities. A similar set of pressures has been brought to bear on local authorities, which have been encouraged to relinquish their role as direct providers of services in favour of a commissioning or 'enabling' role. Stewart & Stoker (1995) observe that the period 1979–1987 (the first two terms of the Thatcher government) saw some 40 Acts of Parliament passed dealing with local government. The outcome of many of these measures and the central thrust of government policy was to increase the control of central government over local authorities and in particular to restrain local authority expenditure.

Chandler (1996) argues that the tradition of local government in Britain is relatively weak compared to other countries in Europe and to the USA. The traditional purposes of local authorities were to spread the administrative load of government, to deliver effective local services and to facilitate pluralist democracy. However, these traditional justifications have been challenged in recent years by what Hill (1994) labels post-Fordist and public choice perspectives. First, post-Fordists such as Stoker (1991) argue that service delivery should be seen as separate from the more important strategic and regulatory functions of local government. A local authority should conceptualize itself as a 'networker', operating in partnership with other local agencies and enterprises to develop local economic and social strategies. The local authority should not be a monolithic provider of services, but should welcome the opportunities for diversity and flexibility which the private and voluntary sectors offer:

> As to the role of the local authority, the network model would give equal weight to service delivery and strategic functions. The former would be carried out by direct provision but also through working with other public, private and voluntary organisations. The latter would express the local authority's concern for issues beyond its statutory responsibilities. The authority would deal, in co-operation with other organisations, with whatever issues were of concern in its area. The network model would support a reform which gave local authorities the power of 'general competence' – the right to act on behalf of their local communities – in addition to the current system of

limited, statutorily-allocated responsibilities. (Stoker 1991, p. 267)

Stoker, professor of politics at the University of Strathclyde, is an influential voice in the debate over the future of local government and his writing has much in common with that of the equally influential John Stewart, professor of local government and administration at the University of Birmingham. Stewart's wife is leader of Birmingham City Council, and Stewart himself is a frequent speaker at Labour Party local government conferences. Stewart (1995) also argues for a power of general competence for local authorities, which would strengthen the local authority's role as 'the community governing itself' (Stewart 1995, p. 252) and advance local government beyond the focus on the direct provision of services. Writers who adopt the post-Fordist perspective, therefore, envisage an enhanced role for local government as the orchestrator of local decision making, economic development and community identity.

This post-Fordist vision of diversity contrasts with the traditional concept of a multi-purpose authority within which services were both planned and delivered (Hill 1994). This traditional approach produced collaborative and cooperative mechanisms within local authorities, but was attacked during the 1980s as too bureaucratic and lacking in accountability to the consumers of services. As in other public enterprises, the Conservative government regarded market competition as necessary to overcome these defects. Informing this position was a public choice theoretical perspective, which emphasized the role of the rational individual who makes informed choices in the market-place. The public choice approach advocated the disbanding of public service monopolies in favour of a market-place of competing providers from the private and not-for-profit sectors. Within public sector institutions, producers should be required to provide for consumer choices through provider–purchaser contracting, performance related rewards and performance appraisal (Hill 1994).

Indeed, direct service provision by local authorities was greatly reduced in the 1980s. Legislation was passed which required the following services to be subjected to compulsory competitive tendering: road repairs, housing repairs, ground maintenance, cleaning, refuse collection, the management of sports and leisure facilities, school meals, the inspection of schools, careers advisory services, housing management services, computing services, legal services and a number of administrative facilities (Blackman 1995). Many Labour-controlled councils successfully kept services in-house by creating more business-like direct service organizations (DSOs) managed separately from council departments representing the 'client'. However, this often occurred at the expense of the terms and conditions of workers employed within the DSOs (Sedgwick-Jell 1996).

The incoming Labour government of 1997 has promised to overturn a number of the quasi-market mechanisms established by its Conservative predecessors, including the internal market in health care. The 1997 government's manifesto also states that it will no longer insist that a council's services should be put out to tender (Labour Party 1997). However, it is likely that policy will develop along the lines of the pluralist approach advocated by the neo-Fordists as opposed to a wholesale return to the direct public provision of services. The need to obtain 'best value' will be emphasized, wherein there will be no preconceptions about who should deliver a service, but where councils will have to demonstrate that their preference is a sound one (Local Government Information Unit 1997). During the 1980s financial controls of central government became extensive, curtailing local expenditure above prescribed central limits by setting targets and penalties and by laying down 'capping' limits to the rates which local authorities could levy. The proportion of local government spending financed by central government rose from 48% in 1980 to over 80% in 1992–3, reinforcing central government control over council spending (Hill 1994). Legislative changes promoted privatization and contracting out, including council house sales, deregulation of municipal public transport and the opting out of schools from local authority control. The 1997 Labour government is committed to undoing many of these changes, but it is likely that the vision of local government as 'enabling' rather than directly providing will remain. The New Labour government is pledged to abolish universal 'capping' and to widen the local tax base, which means local authorities will be given greater financial freedom. However, New Labour has also pledged that there will be no 'excessive' council tax rises, so some mechanism for the centre to retain control over local budgets will have to remain in place.

THE ROLE OF LOCAL AUTHORITIES IN PROMOTING AND MAINTAINING PUBLIC HEALTH

Interestingly, the role of local authorities in promoting and maintaining public health is less open to negotiation than many other aspects of their role. A number of local government services safeguard the health of the public by monitoring environmental hazards and taking enforcement action (Blackman 1995). Such services include: the control of pollution from domestic and industrial sources not governed by the Environmental Agency; enforcing health and safety regulations in the commercial sector; food safety and hygiene; pest control; and the enforcement of trading standards. Local authorities can prosecute traders selling unsafe toys or furniture which does not meet fire regulations. Councils also have the powers to grant or withhold planning permission for new buildings, although the applicants can appeal if they are refused. Councils can impose restrictions on businesses, for example specifying that garages can only work within certain hours. Other important functions include street cleaning and domestic and commercial waste management. Although local authorities are currently compelled to put services such as refuse collection out to tender, they retain overall responsibility for monitoring standards. Local authorities have responsibility for traffic planning and management and can implement strategies to reduce accidents, including traffic calming and the installation of speed cameras.

Origins of local government in public health

Sedgwick-Jell (1996) states that the origins of modern local government lay very much with the concern for public health in the middle of the 19th century. Health authorities were first established by the Public Health Act of 1848 in order to build water purification and sewage systems to eradicate epidemic disease. Rationalization of 19th-century local government was consolidated in an Act of 1894, which used the boundaries of the health boards to create multi-purpose rural and urban district councils. The concern with promoting public health and well-being continued in the first half of the 20th century. Almost one-third of homes erected between the wars were built by local authorities in a building programme aimed at producing 'homes fit for heroes' (Lowry 1991). This period was also characterized by advances in medical care, particularly in maternal and child health services. Local authorities prior to the inception of the National Health Service in 1948 delivered much of what we now consider health care.

Public health and health promotion

Notwithstanding the historical and contemporary importance of local government in maintaining public and environmental health, the concept of 'health' itself is not necessarily high on the local authority agenda. The division of local authorities into a number of discrete departments such as housing or leisure services does not encourage an integrated approach to policy implementation. An important way in which those interested in public health and health promotion can advance healthy public policies, therefore, is through overarching movements such as Healthy Cities and Health for All which have grown from the principles outlined in the Declaration of Alma-Ata (World Health Organization 1978). Within this approach, contemporary health problems are seen to be collective as opposed to individual in origin, and have become the subject of policies dealing with employment, housing, leisure and the environment as well as health care provision (Ashton & Seymour 1988). A number of books have been published which document the successes and the lessons of the Healthy Cities movement (Ashton & Seymour 1988, Ashton 1992, Davies & Kelly 1993). Liverpool, Belfast, Sheffield and Glasgow are examples of UK cities where this approach has enjoyed a high profile and where the concept of the Healthy City has provided a 'banner' for inter-agency working in which local government plays an important role. The UK Health for All movement is more inclusive, recognizing the importance of health promoting policies for rural areas and small towns as well as cities. A particularly good account of the realities of implementing such policies in local government can be found in Allen (1992), who explores the implementation of the Healthy Oxford project.

Global concern

More recently, world governments met to discuss the global environment at the 'earth summit' of 1992, which resulted in the global action plan for sustainable development, Agenda 21. Agenda 21 calls on local authorities throughout the world to develop their own 'Local Agenda 21', and over 200 councils throughout the UK have responded so far (Real World Coalition 1996). In Nottingham, the health authority has taken the lead in drawing up a health strategy entitled Health in your Environment (Nottingham Health Action Group 1997). The strategy includes action points for the different agencies involved in promoting public health (see Fig. 5.2). It will be noted that four of the organizations identified fall within the remit of 'elected' local government, namely housing, environmental health, technical and social services. The Environment Agency and the Health and Safety Executive are agencies of central government who maintain regional and local offices.

Inter-agency working

UK health policy contains a growing emphasis on the importance of inter-agency work. This is captured by the concept of 'healthy alliances' in *The health of the nation* (DOH 1992), where 'local authorities have an important role in promoting public health and are key players with health authorities' (DOH 1992, p. 23). However, it is important not to underestimate the challenge which this agenda presents. It is easy to get carried away by the rhetoric associated with movements such as Health for All, and lose sight of the difficulties in making connections in the real world of hous-

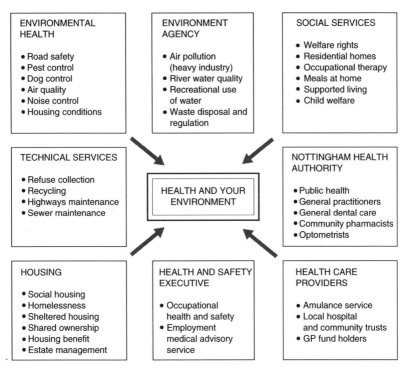

ENVIRONMENTAL
HEALTH

- Road safety
- Pest control
- Dog control
- Air quality
- Noise control
- Housing conditions

ENVIRONMENT
AGENCY

- Air pollution
  (heavy industry)
- River water quality
- Recreational use
  of water
- Waste disposal and
  regulation

SOCIAL SERVICES

- Welfare rights
- Residential homes
- Occupational therapy
- Meals at home
- Supported living
- Child welfare

TECHNICAL SERVICES

- Refuse collection
- Recycling
- Highways maintenance
- Sewer maintenance

HEALTH AND YOUR
ENVIRONMENT

NOTTINGHAM HEALTH
AUTHORITY

- Public health
- General practitioners
- General dental care
- Community pharmacists
- Optometrists

HOUSING

- Social housing
- Homelessness
- Sheltered housing
- Shared ownership
- Housing benefit
- Estate management

HEALTH AND SAFETY
EXECUTIVE

- Occupational
  health and safety
- Employment
  medical advisory
  service

HEALTH CARE
PROVIDERS

- Amulance service
- Local hospital
  and community trusts
- GP fund holders

Fig. 5.2 Agencies involved in promoting public health in Nottingham (after Nottingham Health Action Group, Nottingham Health Authority 1997, with permission).

ing offices and health centres. For example, Conway (1995) outlines the key role of housing as an instrument of health care, quoting Florence Nightingale: 'The connection between health and the dwellings of the population is one of the most important that exists' (Nightingale 1860, cited in Conway 1995, p. 141).

However, a recent report exploring the quality of inter-agency working between housing and health services concluded that there are many barriers to successful collaboration, not least due to the introduction of quasi-markets in health and social care:

> *The introduction of competition tends to lead to a narrow, specialist approach to services, and to increased separation of agencies. This does not encourage an integrated holistic approach to service provision. The emphasis on making agencies more "accountable" for their performance tends to focus agencies on narrow indicators, which do not reward collaboration or support long-term goals. (Arblaster et al 1996, p. ix).*

In a climate of restricted resources, it is important that inter-agency working to promote ideals such as Health for All is not seen as a solution to the grossly uneven distribution of wealth which results in persistent and widening inequalities in health (Wilkinson 1996). However, by adopting proactive policies to address poverty, local government is in a position to do much to improve the quality of life for its citizens and to promote the public's health.

THE ROLE OF LOCAL AUTHORITY PRACTITIONERS IN THE PERSONAL SOCIAL SERVICES

The health of the nation (DOH 1992) acknowledges that local authorities contribute to health through the purchasing and direct provision of social services as well as through their role in public health. The drive towards primary care led health services is increasing the emphasis on collaboration between health and social services, as the White Paper *Primary care: delivering the future* makes clear (DOH 1996). However, both health and social services are experiencing pressures which make such collaboration problematic. Historically, services provided by the NHS are free at the point of delivery whereas social services are means tested. As both services experience funding shortages, so the debate as to what constitutes health and what social care intensifies (Prail 1997). Recent research by Twigg (1997) illustrates the very real implications of this debate for older people who need help with bathing, for whom the question 'is it a "medical" or a "social" bath?' has important consequences. Other authors have suggested that community care policies are not meeting their stated aim of promoting service users' choice and dignity but are actually accelerating gaps in service provision (Richardson & Pearson 1995). At the other end of the lifespan, well publicized enquiries into the abuse and deaths of children 'at risk' have highlighted the dangers of inadequate communication between health and social care agencies. The Children Act of 1989 was designed to overcome some of the conflicts and ambiguities which characterized childcare work in the 1980s, again emphasizing the importance of inter-agency cooperation. However, there is evidence that the different professions contributing to health and social care have quite distinct occupational cultures. Pietroni (1996) evaluated a programme of inter-professional training involving nursing, medical and social work students. He found that each group of students had powerful and often negative stereotypes of the work of the others, which provides a possible explanation of why teamwork is so difficult. Perhaps one important factor is the lack of understanding among health care professionals of the climate in which their colleagues in local government operate. Also, the historical and contemporary influences which shape the development of the professions may lead to different values and priorities. For example, social workers have traditionally placed more emphasis on issues associated with equal opportunities than their colleagues in health.

Social services departments are actually a fairly recent phenomenon. In England and Wales they were created by the

Local Authority Social Services Act of 1970 and in Scotland by the Social Work (Scotland) Act of 1968. In the 2 decades from 1970 to 1990, their importance to local government grew rapidly as the proportion of local government revenue expenditure devoted to the personal social services doubled. Willis (1995) suggests a number of reasons for this growth:

• Every aspect of social services practice was subjected to major legislative change, with the net effect of increasing the duties and responsibilities of social services departments.

• The consumer population of social services departments increased dramatically, including a 50% rise in the number of people over 85. Greater awareness of the prevalence of child abuse, and the development of community-based mental health services also contributed to a growth in consumer demand, as did the rise in unemployment and the widening disparity between the earnings of the rich and the poor.

• Public enquiries into scandals affecting both children and adults pushed social services to the forefront of political and public debate and increased the workload associated with inspection and regulation.

Adams (1996) highlights the further changes that have accompanied the development of quasi-markets in social care in the 1990s. Public choice perspectives suggest that the users of services are customers who can exercise rational choice over which services to access. The vision of the 'enabling authority' applies just as much to the functioning of social services departments as to other departments within local government. The community care reforms, in particular, required social services departments to spend 85% of their community care budgets outside the public sector. In contrast to the 'internal market' in the NHS, the separation of the purchasing and providing functions in the personal social services has been used as a device to stimulate the independent and not-for-profit sectors (Glendenning 1996).

Community care

The drive to contain costs appears to be having a detrimental impact on the ability of the community care reforms to realize their potential. A report published by the National Association of Citizens' Advice Bureaux (1997), *Rationing community care*, claims that financial pressures on local authorities are forcing them to concentrate their resources on those with the most pressing needs. Basic services such as shopping, bathing and cleaning are being withdrawn. In 1997, Gloucestershire County Council withdrew home care services from 1500 disabled people following a £2.5 million cut in funding, and an appeal failed to get the services reinstated. Certainly, some of the new directions associated with 'the enabling authority' have increased personal choice, for example in allowing people with disabilities to manage their own budget when purchasing services to meet their needs. However, the strict cash limits applied to local authority spending suggest the metaphor of the user as consumer of personal social services is limited.

Children and families

Aspects of social services work relating to children and families has been less susceptible to the 'enabling' philosophy because much of the work carried out in this area is of a statutory nature. However, underfunding is also a serious problem in work with families, forcing social workers to concentrate on issues of child protection rather than the preventive work which may prove more fruitful in the long term. Baldock (1994) argues that the evolution of the personal social services has been led neither by assessment of need nor by response to demand. Instead, the allocation of resources has been determined by the wheeling and dealing which goes on in the process of setting the budgets for the different departments of local government. This process was starkly illustrated in an exercise carried out by Nottinghamshire County Council entitled *Opening the books*. Faced with severe cuts in the centrally allocated budget, councillors asked the public themselves to choose priorities, for example between fire services and community care or between education and child protection. Unfortunately, there is little indication that the incoming Labour government of 1997 will commit further resources to the personal social services, so it is likely that such political priority setting exercises will continue to be necessary.

LOCAL GOVERNMENT AND THE DEBATE OVER CITIZENSHIP

From the 1970s onwards elements of the left, right and centre of the political spectrum have increasingly challenged the belief that the established form of local government is capable of solving social and economic problems (Stewart & Stoker 1995). In response, the changes in local government of the 1980s and 1990s have been the subject of debate not only over specific provisions – over finance, functions, structure and management – but also over the role which local government should play in the modern state (Hill 1994). The debate has focused on the role of local authorities as 'enablers' as well as 'providers' of services. Much has been made of 'empowering' people to make choices, whether as citizens through participation in and access to local government, or as consumers through the redress and influence offered by market-provided services.

Arguments have also continued as to the appropriate size of local authorities in terms of size, function and possibilities for effective participation. Hill (1994) argues that local government must be accountable to its electorate as a community of citizens, not just to consumers concerned with individual redress. The essential feature of local government is that the wider public interest is represented by the body of elected councillors, who should assess local needs and problems and evaluate the effectiveness of service delivery on behalf of local people. Elections, in turn, give dissatisfied voters the opportunity to reject their representatives and elect someone else. However, because local government is run on party political lines, it is possible for ineffective councillors to continue in office simply because they continue to stand for re-election on the party slate. It should also be noted that the United Kingdom has one of the highest ratios of electors to councillors of any country in Europe, about 1 councillor to every 2200 citizens compared to 1 to 325 in similar Western states (Hill 1994). Councillors may claim to be in touch with local people but only just over 20% of the electorate will have contacted a councillor in the last 5 years (Stewart 1995). Such sobering statistics have encouraged a wide-ranging debate over ways of increasing participation in the processes of local government. Pratchett & Wilson (1997) review the report of the independent Commission for Local Democracy (CLD) established in 1993. The CLD recommend extending the role of local government to become more active champions of local democracy and active citizenship. 'Citizenship' should become part of the national curriculum in schools and mechanisms for direct consultation and citizen involvement in decision making should be established. Such thinking is very much in tune with the New Labour project to strengthen civil society. In a review of the challenges posed by the New Labour agenda, Filkin (1997) calls for changes in the role of local government which will:

- develop a new, positive role for local councils of community leadership, with new powers and responsibilities to pursue the public interest

- promote democratic renewal through new ways of working with the general public, involving them in the council's processes as well as raising electoral turnout

- develop political leadership and experiment with new political systems

- deliver best value for the public, aiming to improve efficiency and effectiveness of services and to deal with service failures quickly and openly

- improve the 'fit' between the objectives of central government, local government and what local communities want, particularly in relation to crime, education, employment, health and the environment.

A system of local government revitalized according to the principles outlined above would indeed have the potential to increase participation in decision making for both individual citizens and communities.

Despite the difficulties in claiming to be truly representative, most councillors pride themselves on their accessibility to individuals and groups within their localities. Many establish regular advice 'surgeries' held at familiar venues such as libraries or community centres, and councillors' home telephone numbers are circulated on leaflets and posters. The important point here is that nurses and other health care workers can influence the policy making process by lobbying local councillors over issues of concern. Such issues could include individual clients' problems, for example where there is a need for the councillor to act as advocate with the housing department. Health workers can also work with the local authority on events such as 'national no smoking day', where leisure centres may be willing participants in health promotion activities. It is possible to move such concerns onto the wider agenda of towns and cities, for example by staging a seminar on a particular topic and inviting elected members and council officers to attend. Sometimes nurses will find themselves in an oppositional position to the local authority, for example over the planned closure of residential homes or schools. This is still part of the process of active participation in local democracy, and nurses should be prepared to make their case. According to Wass (1994), the nurse's role in promoting health includes both working with communities (community development) and working for communities. The community development approach involves assessing health needs, encouraging public participation, providing resources and assisting community members in skills development and research. Working for communities, on the other hand, implies contributing to healthy public policy through advocacy and lobbying at local and national levels. As individual citizens, too, nurses can exercise their right to get involved in local political parties, to question candidates during elections and to continue the dialogue through participation in public meetings and debate.

CONCLUSION

This chapter has endeavoured to convey a sense of both the historical development of local government and of contemporary debates over its structure and function. The role of local government in promoting public health and in providing (or 'enabling') the personal social services has been explored. It is hoped the reader will realize that local government does have significance in British politics, not least because it is the most accessible point for active participation in political activity. Local authorities are responsible not only for the direct provision of services, but also for creating a climate in which individuals and communities can prosper. As anyone engaged in promoting health and well-being knows, this can be an uphill struggle. Local government is operating in the same climate as nurses and the National Health Service, where it is expected that efficiency savings will continue to be made year after year. However, even in an economic climate of cuts and retrenchment we can take heart from the examples of good practice and innovative planning underpinning local government throughout the UK. Central government may hold the purse strings but there is – even today – space for elected councillors and local government officers to shape the services nurses and their clients rely on.

■ **QUESTIONS FOR DISCUSSION**

- How did local government develop in the UK?
- What is the role of local authorities in promoting and maintaining public health?
- How do people get elected as councillors?
- How can nurses and other health workers bring the needs of patients and clients to the attention of local councillors and thus onto the local policy agenda?
- Are you aware of any 'healthy alliances' between your health authority and local authority? If so, are nurses involved?
- What does the vision of an 'enabling' local authority suggest for the future of community care?

Cont'd

■ **QUESTIONS FOR DISCUSSION** (*cont'd*)

- How effective is local government in promoting active citizenship and democratic participation in your local community?
- How effective and efficient are your local authority's services?

FURTHER READING

Allen P 1992 Off the rocking horse: how local councils can promote your health and environment. Green Print, London

The author is an environmental health officer with Oxford City Council, and the book is an account of the Healthy Oxford project. It is written in a lively, accessible style and is full of practical examples of ways in which local alliances can be forged to promote public health.

Blackman T 1995 Urban policy in practice. Routledge, London

This book offers a comprehensive guide to urban policy, which addresses the contemporary priorities of sustainable development, social and economic regeneration and effective service delivery. The book is densely written and rather complex, but contains an excellent chapter on 'Health for All' which could be read in isolation by anyone interested in promoting health in cities.

Chandler J 1996 Local government today, 2nd edn. Manchester University Press, Manchester

An up-to-date book which gives a clear and concise account of the processes of local government in the UK. This text provides an insight into the key issues affecting local government, and has a particularly good chapter on the functions of local authorities, including those related to public health.

Hill D 1994 Citizens and cities: urban policy in the 1990s. Harvester Wheatsheaf, London

This book explores key issues affecting people's quality of life in cities, including crime, racism and social exclusion. This book is recommended to anyone who wants to get to grips with the philosophical and political dilemmas associated with realizing citizenship through local democracy.

Wilson D, Game C 1994 Local government in the United Kingdom. Macmillan, Basingstoke

An ideal book for anyone who is interested in standing for election to a local authority or who is interested in finding out more about local government. This book covers a broad range of topics and is presented in a lively and accessible format. The text is informed by 'real life' examples, which keep the reader engaged, and the authors do not shy away from some of the more controversial issues in town hall politics.

REFERENCES

Adams R 1996 The personal social services: clients, consumers or citizens? Longman, London

Allen P 1992 Off the rocking horse: how local councils can promote your health and environment. Green Print, London

Arblaster L, Conway J, Foreman A, Hawtin M 1996 Asking the impossible: inter-agency working to address the housing, health and social care needs of people in ordinary housing. Policy Press, University of Bristol, Bristol

Ashton J (ed) 1992 Healthy cities. Open University Press, Milton Keynes

Ashton J, Seymour H 1988 The new public health. Open University Press, Milton Keynes

Baldock J 1994 The personal social services: the politics of care. In: George V, Miller S (eds) Social policy towards 2000: squaring the welfare circle. Routledge, London, ch 8, pp 161–189

Blackman T 1995 Urban policy in practice. Routledge, London

Byrne T 1994 Local government in Britain, 6th edn. Penguin, London

Chandler J 1996 Local government today, 2nd edn. Manchester University Press, Manchester

Cochrane A 1992 Is there a future for local government? Critical Social Policy 35:4–19

Cole M, Boyne G 1995 So you think you know what local government is? Local Government Studies 21(2):191–202

Conway J 1995 Housing as an instrument of health care. Health and Social Care in the Community 3:141–150

Davies J, Kelly M 1993 Healthy cities: research and practice. Routledge, London

Department of Health 1992 The health of the nation: a strategy for health in England. HMSO, London

Department of Health 1996 Primary care: delivering the future. HMSO, London

Filkin G 1997 Transformation and democracy. Local Government Chronicle Issue no. 6752(9 May 1997):16–17

Glendenning C 1996 The changing interface between primary care and social care. In: Boyd R (ed) What is the future for a primary care-led NHS? National Primary Care Research and Development Centre/Radcliffe Medical Press, Oxford, pp 45–52

Hill D 1994 Citizens and cities: urban policy in the 1990s. Harvester Wheatsheaf, London

Labour Party 1997 New Labour: because Britain deserves better [1997 Manifesto]. Labour Party, London

Le Grand J 1997 Knight, knaves or pawns? Human behaviour and social policy. Journal of Social Policy 26(2):149–169

Local Government Information Unit 1997 A new start? LGIU Briefing 107(May):6–11

Lowry S 1991 Housing and health. British Medical Journal Publishing, London

National Association of Citizens' Advice Bureaux 1997 Rationing community care. National Association of Citizens' Advice Bureaux, London

Nottingham Health Action Group 1997 Health in your environment. Nottingham Health Authority, Nottingham

Pietroni P 1996 Innovation in community care and primary health. Churchill Livingstone, Edinburgh

Prail M 1997 A bumpy ride for pilot schemes. Health Service Journal 107:15

Pratchett L, Wilson D 1997 The rebirth of local democracy? Local Government Studies 23(1):16–31

Real World Coalition 1996 The politics of the real world. Earthscan, London

Richardson S, Pearson M 1995 Dignity and aspirations denied: unmet health and social care needs in an inner-city area. Health and Social Care in the Community 3(5):279–287

Royal College of Nursing 1992 The value of nursing. RCN, London

Sedgwick-Jell S 1996 Local authorities servicing health: rediscovering an historic role. In: Bywaters P, McLeod E (eds) Working for equality in health. Routledge, London, ch 8, pp 117–123

Stewart J 1995 A future for local authorities as community government. In: Stewart J, Stoker G (eds) Local government in the 1990s. Macmillan, Basingstoke, ch 14, pp 249–267

Stewart J, Stoker G (eds) 1995 Local government in the 1990s. Macmillan, Basingstoke

Stoker G 1991 The politics of local government. Macmillan, Basingstoke

Twigg J 1997 Deconstructing the 'social bath': help with bathing at home for older and disabled people. Journal of Social Policy 26(2):211–232

Walker D 1996 A place for trust: local government and the people. Local Government Information Unit, London

Wass A 1994 Promoting health: the primary health care approach. W B Saunders/Baillière Tindall, Sydney

Wilkinson R 1996 Unhealthy societies: the afflictions of inequality. Routledge, London

Willis M 1995 Community care and social services. In: Stewart J, Stoker G (eds) Local government in the 1990s. Macmillan, Basingstoke, ch 8, pp 126–144

Wilson D, Game C 1994 Local government in the United Kingdom. Macmillan, Basingstoke

World Health Organization 1978 Declaration of Alma-Ata. Reproduced in: Wass A 1994 Promoting health: the primary health care approach. W B Saunders/Baillière Tindall, Sydney, pp 217–219

Parliament, UK politics and the European Union

Jean S. Neave

■ **CONTENTS**

INTRODUCTION

Nursing is shaped by the social, economic and political forces within the United Kingdom and by events internationally, particularly in Europe. The directions, goals and principles of government have continually influenced nursing in the UK. Often nurses fail to acknowledge that their work exists within a wider context which controls and rations the resources that support the health care system, ultimately affecting what nursing is and the way in which nursing care is delivered. The European Union (EU) was created with the aim of securing lasting peace and cooperation in Europe. With the gradual moves towards European integration and the growth in membership the EU has had an increasing influence on all of our lives. Not only do we have the freedom to travel and seek work in any EU country, but also European directives have agreed common standards that have directly influenced the content of nursing and midwifery education. Member states are encouraged to cooperate on joint public health programmes and exchange information and good practice with other European colleagues. Nursing in the UK seeks to influence European policy making on health issues in order to benefit nurses and improve patient/client care.

The aim of this chapter is to stimulate in nurses an interest and awareness of the fundamental importance and relevance of the British government and the EU to their everyday practice. The chapter is divided into two parts. In the first part I will examine the role of Parliament in the UK. In the second I will move on to examine the UK and its place in Europe.

REGISTRATION OF THE PROFESSIONS

From the late 19th century midwives and nurses campaigned vigorously for registration of their professions by the state. They were determined to achieve registration to improve the standards of their professions and thereby give a better and higher standard of service to the public. Midwives and nurses also acknowledged that registration would enhance status. The opposition they faced was enormous, especially at the beginning of their campaigns when the medical profession opposed registration, but the nurses and midwives persisted. Registration of midwives was achieved in 1902 but it was not until after the First World War that registration of nurses was achieved (1919). The government had to present the Bill because of bitter disagreement between rival nursing organizations. The General Nursing Council was established in 1920 (Hart 1994). The relationship between Parliament and nursing is close because the profession is regulated by statute. Any major changes to nursing, midwifery and health visiting have to be approved by Parliament. It is important, therefore, that nurses understand the political process within the Houses of Parliament in order that they can influence this process.

DEMOCRACY AND THE CONSTITUTION

The British form of government is based on the principle of representative democracy; the electorate is given the opportunity to vote at least every 5 years to decide who will represent them in the House of Commons. The term 'democracy' means rule by the 'demos' – the people – and in the British system of government, members of the House of Commons are given the right to rule only because they have been elected by a majority. A common definition of democracy is 'government of the people, by the people, for the people' and most theorists would agree that a democratic form of government should satisfy three elements:

- government of the people means that a democracy only has power over its own citizens

- government by the people implies that there is a collective system by which people rule, not a single person

- government for the people describes a system where the government is in power for the sake of the citizens, not the rulers (Wolff 1996).

Democracy is also seen to embody the values of freedom and equality. Freedom consists of giving people a say in decision making and particularly in those decisions that affect them. Equality is embodied by giving the right of decision making to all. There has been much discussion recently about the democratic nature of our institutions of government; Charter 88 is a pressure group which has campaigned for a modern and fair democracy.

One way it is proposed to give people more direct control is to allow the electorate to participate in referenda on important matters, especially those involving changes to the constitution, for example devolution in Scotland and Wales (the pros and cons of devolution will be addressed later in the chapter). However, in exercising one's individual rights there is a challenge to the sovereignty of Parliament and a tension between the rights of the majority and the minority. Prior to joining the European Community (EC) in the early 1970s the UK had a sovereign British Parliament, where laws were made by Parliament and enforced by the state. Since becoming a member of the EC, Parliament must refrain from passing legislation which contradicts European law. This is seen as eroding the ability of Parliament to govern and make legislation on behalf of the nation. This loss of sovereignty continues to concern many politicians, for example the Eurosceptics in the various political parties.

It is not only because of the relationship nursing has with Parliament that knowledge of the constitution is important to nurses. Dearlove & Saunders (1991) suggest three further reasons why a study of the constitution is important.

• The established constitution operates on politics and provides a constraining and enabling context within which much political activity occurs (for example it regulates public access to, and the behaviour of, various institutions and officials and enforces a general election every 5 years).

• The constitution is frequently a political issue in its own right (for instance, the Labour government elected in 1997 is committed to making the system of government more open and democratic (Labour Party 1997)).

• Constitutional theory is about politics itself: it provides us with a perspective on the location of power, the structure of relationships between the state and organizations and associations, such as pressure groups, in society.

Parliament is the supreme legislative authority in Britain. Unlike most other countries, parliamentary government is not based on a written constitution, although it is one of the oldest representative assemblies. It is composed of three components: the monarch, the House of Lords and the House of Commons. Agreement by all three has to be obtained for legislation to be passed.

THE MONARCH

The legal existence of Parliament depends upon the exercise of the royal prerogative, which is the collection of residual powers left in the hands of the Crown (COI 1994). Most of these powers are now exercised on behalf of others or on the advice of ministers and are governed by convention. Among the 'powers' which still remain within the royal prerogative are the choosing of the prime minister, the assent to legislation, the dispensing of ministerial portfolios and the dissolution of Parliament (Jones et al 1991).

THE HOUSE OF LORDS

The House of Lords consists of the lords spiritual, hereditary peers, law lords and life peers. Hereditary peers form the largest group and consequently there is an in-built Conservative Party bias. The potential membership is about 1200, but many hereditary peers do not attend. The House of Lords is presided over by the lord chancellor, who is appointed by the prime minister and also has a seat in the Cabinet.

According to Birch (1993), the House of Lords has four main functions:

1. Members question ministers about the activities of the government and stage debates on general issues of national policy.

2. The House of Lords saves House of Commons time. They can give first readings to non-controversial Bills which subsequently pass through the Commons with little discussion. Since 1945, 25% of all Bills have been dealt with in this way. These are mainly technical Bills, for example those concerned with company law.

3. The House of Lords can revise details of Bills. Much more legislation is being introduced in the House of Commons each session and consequently there is not enough time to

discuss it all thoroughly. The more detailed consideration of legislation afforded in the Lords is welcomed by organizations representing interests likely to be affected by the legislation. Health visitors, district nurses and midwives used this opportunity to express their concerns about some aspects of the Nurses, Midwives and Health Visitors Bill 1979.

4. The most controversial function of the House of Lords is that it may reject Bills from the House of Commons, although increasingly the power of the Lords to veto Bills has been restricted and ignored.

The House of Lords has lost its former historical position in Parliament because it is not an elected chamber and has no power. However, it has legal authority and is still the final court of appeal for civil cases in Britain and for criminal cases in England, Wales and Northern Ireland.

It is anticipated that the House of Lords and Houses of Parliament will be reformed, although the legislative jurisdiction of the House of Lords will remain (Labour Party 1997).

Lord Jenkins, former chief of the Liberal Democrats, was appointed by Tony Blair in December 1997 to head an electoral reform commission. The Cabinet will examine any recommendations made and the public will decide, in a referendum, whether to change the voting system. In 1969, however, a Bill to reform the House of Lords had to be withdrawn because of extreme hostility from both government and the opposition party (Birch 1993).

THE HOUSE OF COMMONS

The House of Commons, most recently elected in May 1997,

is composed of 659 members of parliament, the largest number since 1918. The UK is divided into geographical parliamentary constituencies. Boundary Commissions, who base their decisions primarily on shifts in the population, determine the number of constituencies.

MPs are elected by secret ballot, using the first-past-the-post system. The candidate who receives the largest number of votes is the person elected. British citizens over 18 years of age are entitled to vote, but individuals have to be registered in the current electoral register. This is prepared annually by the electoral registration officers of the local authority (COI 1994). It is important that nurses, who move residences frequently, maintain their electoral registration. There are some groups of people who are not entitled to vote; these include members of the House of Lords and patients detained under mental health legislation. In 1997 voter turnout was 71.4%, which was a fall of 7% compared to the 1992 general election. This figure has caused concern and there had been discussion before the 1997 general election, and since, about changing the electoral system to a form of proportional representation. The present system tends to disadvantage third and other parties (see Ch. 3 where Dearlove and Taggart discuss representative government in greater depth).

MPs should represent all their constituents collectively; if a constituent has a problem with a government policy, department or public service they can contact their MP. MPs are also lobbied by professional organizations and trade unions (see Ch. 4 for Cameron's exploration of the role of interest groups in the political process).

The political party which has the largest number of MPs forms the government and it is their primary duty to maintain the government in power. MPs have three principal functions: the first is give their assent, or otherwise, to legislation which has been brought before the House of Commons; the second function is to take part in debates; and the third is to scrutinize the actions of the government. This can be performed by scrutiny of proposed legislation. Executive actions can also be considered by debate or by raising constituency problems, resulting from executive actions, at parliamentary questions. MPs can be elected onto select committees, which are specifically formed to examine, for instance, the expenditure, administration and policy of principal government departments. For example Ann Keen MP, one of the first nurses to become an MP, elected in 1997, sits on the select committee for health. MPs also correspond with ministers on behalf of constituents, raise matters of concern on the floor of the House and can table an Early Day Motion (Jones et al 1991).

THE LAW MAKING PROCESS

Fundamental changes to the law are ultimately the responsibility of Parliament and the government. A minister of the government or a 'backbencher' MP can introduce public Bills into either the House of Lords or House of Commons. Government Bills are usually introduced in the House of Commons, especially those which might be controversial. Bills are drafted by civil servants for the minister responsible. Bills usually have the approval of the Cabinet before ministers present them to Parliament.

Before government Bills are introduced, Green Papers (consultation papers) may be prepared which set out government proposals which are still under consideration. At this stage, comments are requested from people, or groups, who have an interest in or may be affected by the proposals. If the proposals affect nursing, for example, statutory bodies, professional organizations, trade unions and individuals can present their opinions. These bodies may also have lobbied and requested the proposed legislation. White Papers are statements of government intent and may be issued by the government for consultation before a Bill is introduced. For example *Working for patients*, which announced many of the changes to the NHS which were formalized in the NHS and Community Care Act 1990, was introduced as a White Paper in 1989 (DOH 1989).

When a Bill is introduced it has to go through three readings, a committee and a report stage. The first reading consists of a formal introduction. The second reading takes the form of a debate on the main principles of the Bill, but detailed discussion and amendments do not take place until the next stage, the committee stage. It is at this stage that the Bill will be examined by a standing committee of MPs, reflecting the proportions of parties in the House of Commons. Thus, discussion in the committee stage tends to follow party lines. Changes may be made provided that these are in keeping with the main principles of the Bill. After the committee stage the Bill returns to the House of Commons for the report stage. MPs are given an opportunity to speak on the Bill and amendments can be made. The third reading occurs when the House of Commons gives its final approval to the Bill. After the third reading the Bill is sent to the House of Lords and, if any amendments are made, the Bill returns to the House of Commons and any Lords' amendments are debated. When a Bill has completed all its stages in Parliament it is sent to the monarch for royal assent (COI 1994).

It is possible for groups to influence the legislative process as a Bill proceeds through these stages. For example, the Nurses, Midwives and Health Visitors Bill 1979 was delayed because midwives, district nurses and health visitors wanted more recognition of their different traditions. As a consequence health visitors gained separate recognition in the United Kingdom Central Council, and the National Boards' committee structure (Clay 1987).

PRIVATE MEMBERS' BILLS

At the beginning of each session of Parliament, private members of the Commons (that is MPs without Cabinet positions) draw lots for the opportunity to introduce a Bill on one of the Fridays specifically allocated for this purpose. Only 20 MPs will be successful. Private members' Bills are not always debated and many proceed no further than a second reading due to limited parliamentary time. Specific policy areas are usually more successful in private members' Bills, and they may be allowed to lapse or be withdrawn if the government agrees to introduce legislation at a later date or to set up an inquiry (Jones et al 1991). The Royal College of Nursing (RCN) in 1991 approached one of the MPs on its parliamentary panel to present a private members' Bill for the introduction of nurse prescribing. The Bill failed due to lack of government support. However, in 1992 the RCN approached another MP and this time the private members' Bill was successfully negotiated through the legislative process and the Medicinal Products Prescription by Nurses Act was given royal assent in 1992 (Jones & Gough 1997).

STATUTORY INSTRUMENTS

In each session of Parliament an increasing amount of legislation is passed and there is also an increase in the number of legislative orders and regulations which need parliamentary approval. Ministers add, and when necessary change details after an Act has been passed. The principles of the Act have to remain unchanged. These rules and orders are called 'statutory instruments'. The procedure is for them to be laid on the tables of the two Houses of Parliament. They become law unless either of the Houses passes a motion to reject them. Statutory instruments have been used by the Department of Health to make changes to legislation affecting nursing, for example the new rules relating to nurse training in 1983, changes to the UKCC voting rules, and in defining the class of nurse empowered to detain a patient under Section 5 (4) of the Mental Health Act 1983.

THE CABINET

The rising control of political parties in the House of Commons has changed the relationship between the Cabinet and the House of Commons, and has resulted in the increasing dominance of the prime minister and the Cabinet. There are usually 20 members of the Cabinet and the secretary of state for health usually has a place in the Cabinet. Cabinet ministers are chosen by the prime minister, who chairs Cabinet meetings and determines the agenda. The prime minister used to be described as the 'primus inter pares' – the first among equals – but as leader of the political party in control of the House of Commons the power of the prime minister has grown with the rise of the dominance of the political parties in Parliament. The prime minister has considerable power too in making other ministerial appointments, which now amount to over 100. The Prime Minister's power is also manifested by the amount of media coverage given to him. The prime minister is free of departmental responsibilities but has his own office and responsibilities and can add or remove ministerial responsibilities. He also has the power to instruct the Civil Service over the conduct of business, although civil servants are expected to be politically neutral. There is a large network of Cabinet committees, and because the public does not always know of their existence they are protected from lobbying and influence. The chairmanship, composition and powers of committees are the responsibility of the prime minister. Their existence has been seen to weaken the role of the Cabinet, whose members are expected to take collective responsibility for decision making. However, the Cabinet may not always be aware of committee decisions. The prime minister needs allies in order to implement policy and is therefore dependent on the support of colleagues. The prime minister has to balance different views with the party and may have to appoint colleagues who hold alternative views. However, the prime minister may promote and develop colleagues who actively support the party line, even at the expense of demoting or dismissing experienced or more senior colleagues who are less inclined to toe the party line (Dearlove and Saunders 1991).

THE DEPARTMENT OF HEALTH

The health secretary is accountable to Parliament for health and the services provided by local authorities for community care. These include services provided by social services departments, such as services for children and young families, services for older people and services for people with disabilities. There are three ministers of state for health, although this number can vary; for example the Labour government in 1997 introduced a minister specifically responsible for public health. The National Health Service

(NHS) ostensibly is run under the aegis of the National Health Service Executive, located in Leeds, with eight regional offices, but considerable powers have been retained by the DOH and the DOH is exclusively responsible for legislation. The secretary of state for health can intervene in the work of NHS trusts by appointing individuals to trust boards. However, there has been a considerable shift of power from the health authorities, with elected members, to managers of NHS trusts, and officials on the new central and regulatory bodies. The trusts are seen as new QUANGOs (quasi-autonomous non-governmental organizations) which operate at 'arm's length from ministers'. The DOH appoints the chairs of trusts and oversees all appointments and so has substantial powers of patronage. In addition, there are executive bodies which perform their functions under statute. An example is the United Kingdom Central Council for Nursing, Midwifery and Health Visiting (UKCC). This body is responsible for maintaining the professional register and setting standards of education and conduct. Although the majority of UKCC members are elected, one third are appointed by the DOH, to include consumer groups, doctors and lay members. JM Consulting is undertaking a review of the UKCC and the national boards on behalf of the four UK health departments. This was due to report in the summer of 1998 and may result in new legislation that significantly changes the regulation of the professions. Advisory bodies also meet regularly under the aegis of the DOH. These include the standing nursing and midwifery advisory committee.

There is increasing recognition by the government in the UK, and by the DOH, that a stronger public health focus is required in health policy. This is reflected in the appointment of a new minister for public health (Tessa Jowell at the time of publication). The consultative Green Paper, *Our healthier nation* (DOH 1998) focuses on improving the health of the nation as a whole and improving the health of the worst off in society through the establishment of healthy schools, healthy workplaces and healthy neighbourhoods. The paper has reduced the targets from *Health of the nation* (DOH 1992) to four priority areas: heart disease and stroke, accidents, cancer and mental health.

DEVOLUTION

Devolution is the process of transferring power from central government to a lower or regional level. Devolving power to regional level is in keeping with broader political trends across Europe. Both Scotland and Wales have long had devolved administrations – the Scottish Office dates from 1885 and the Welsh Office from 1951. Scotland also has its own legal and educational systems. In June 1997 a guillotine motion, setting a timetable for passage of the Referendum Bill, was passed. In September 1997 the people of Scotland and Wales voted in favour of extended devolution. The arrangements will be different in both Scotland and Wales.

The Scottish Parliament will have 129 members and more powers than the Welsh Assembly. For example the Scottish Parliament will have short term borrowing powers and be able to vary the basic rate of income tax by 3% in order to raise revenue to support its policies. Elections will take place in 1999. The Welsh Assembly will have the power to debate and make recommendations to the secretary of state on any matter relating to Wales. It will take over responsibility for the existing budget of the Welsh Office and its functions.

Defence and foreign policy will remain the responsibility of the UK government. The Scottish White Paper makes a strong restatement of the sovereignty of the Westminster Parliament and underlines the fact that Scotland is being offered devolution not independence. The Queen will continue to be head of state of the UK.

There are many arguments for and against devolution. Supporters argue that devolution will allow political decisions to be more sensitive to the specific needs of the local population. For example supporters of the Welsh Assembly noted that much existing Welsh legislation was passed on a majority of English Conservative MPs. They see the Welsh Assembly as offering the people of Wales more say in the policies which affect them and, conversely, making politicians more accountable for the decisions they take. Opponents, however, have argued that too much government will result in overlapping responsibilities causing confusion, inefficiency and unnecessary administrative costs. For example the running costs of the Scottish Parliament are anticipated to be £20–30 million per annum, which is equivalent to £5 per head of the Scottish population. There is also the point – first raised in the 1970s by Tam Dalyell, Labour MP for West Lothian and therefore known as 'the West Lothian question' – that devolution still lets Scottish MPs at Westminster continue to have a say in English affairs, whilst denying English MPs a vote in Scottish affairs. There are fears that devolution will weaken the UK's voice in Europe and concern that friction will occur, particularly between Edinburgh and Westminster, which might even result in the break-up of the UK.

It is too early to say what the eventual consequences will be for health and nursing. Certainly devolution may allow health policies and priorities to be more sensitive to local needs and local problems. However, there have always been differences in health spending per capita and health policy direction between the four countries of the UK. For example NHS continuing care facilities for older people are still being built in Scotland whereas in most of England all continuing care occurs in the private and independent sector. Nevertheless, the Scottish Parliament could use its tax raising powers to invest more proportionately in health. It is likely that regulation of nurses will remain a UK function although the presence of the new regulatory body may be strengthened in the four countries. There has always been different post-registration provision for continuing education across Scotland, England, Northern Ireland and Wales even though standards and regulatory arrangements for entry to the register are the same. It is interesting, nevertheless, that in anticipation of the extra work associated with the Scottish Parliament the RCN has appointed an extra professional officer in its Edinburgh office.

THE UK AND EUROPE

The UK is a member of the EU, the Council of Europe and the World Health Organization (WHO), which has a regional office in Copenhagen, Denmark, with a nursing and midwifery unit. Knowledge of these institutions is important in understanding developments in nursing internationally. Nursing in the UK has been shaped by legislation from the EU. The WHO acts as a catalyst and facilitator for nursing, midwifery and health visiting in Europe through the regional nursing and midwifery unit and also internationally. The WHO Alma-Ata declaration of 1978 laid the foundation for the European targets for 'Health for All', which in turn laid the foundations for the development of the *Health of the nation* (DOH 1992) and *Our healthier nation* (DOH 1998).

THE EUROPEAN COMMUNITY

The UK became a member of the European Community (EC) on 1 January 1973, after a long process of discussion, debate and negotiation. The EC had developed from the European Economic Community (EEC) which came into existence following the Treaty of Rome, 1957. The aim of the treaty was the development of a 'common market' between the states in which there would be freedom of movement of goods, capital, services and people. There were originally six members: Belgium, France, the Federal Republic of Germany, Italy, Luxembourg and the Netherlands. The UK had been invited to join but declined. The EU arose from a desire of political leaders in continental Europe to break with the past and to move away from the destructive forces of nationalism and rivalry, post Second World War, towards a Europe which worked in partnership and shared power. The term EC has become increasingly generalized since then and used particularly by those who want to emphasize that the EC is more than just a financial institution (Wise & Richard 1993).

Ireland and Denmark joined the EC at the same time as the UK, Greece joined in 1981, and Spain and Portugal in 1986. The last countries to become members were Austria, Sweden and Finland in 1995. There are now 15 states in what is now called the European Union (EU) with a population of approximately 370 million people.

Under the terms of the European Communities Act 1972, which was passed as a necessary condition of joining the EC, European regulations and directives take precedence over British law. They thus deprive the British Parliament and British laws of the supremacy they had previously possessed (Birch 1993). Community legislation consists of *regulations*, which are legally binding and directly enforceable laws, made by the Council of the European Union, and *directives*, which are legally binding but are more flexible and allow national governments to draft the precise laws, to take into account the different national traditions and socioeconomic conditions. However, directives are also legally binding and have to be enacted within 2 years (Wise & Gibb 1993). Thus, the entry of the UK into the EC was seen to challenge parliamentary sovereignty. Opinion was divided about membership of the EC, and so a national referendum, the first for the whole country, was held in June 1975 on whether Britain should remain in the European Community. The result was 64.5% in favour.

In 1986, the member states of the EC agreed the Single European Act. This stipulated that an integrated common market should be established by the end of 1992. The Act provided for majority voting on most issues coming before the Council of Ministers. The Single European Act also called for measures to enhance 'social cohesion' within the EC, one consequence of which was the creation of the Social Chapter in 1989, relating to the fundamental rights of workers (Wise & Gibb 1993).

At the heads of government meeting at Maastricht in Holland in 1991 the Maastricht Treaty, calling for greater European unity, was debated. This included an extension of the powers of the European Parliament and a commitment to work towards greater unity in defence and foreign policy. However, the British government was able to negotiate out of two important sections. The first of these was that those countries that met the criteria would adopt a single currency and European Bank. The second was the Social Chapter (Birch 1993).

There was much disagreement in the UK, then and since, at the Conservative government's decision, on the grounds of inequity (why should British employees have less rights than their European counterparts), and much discussion on the 'social costs' of such legislation. The Maastricht Treaty on European union was signed by the member nations in 1992 but the UK maintained her position and negotiated out of the two sections.

The new Labour government, elected in 1997, has honoured its manifesto commitment to sign up to the Social Chapter and the Social Policy agreement. Two directives have been agreed since Maastricht. The first gives workers in multinational companies the right to be informed of corporate changes through works councils. The second, which was to be enforced in June 1998, gives both parents the right to a minimum of 3 months' unpaid leave for childcare; this is in addition to maternity leave. A third directive is in the planning stage. This will give full-time paid employees sick leave, pensions, holidays, staff discounts and share options benefits to all except casually employed part-time workers. Other directives are also expected on minimum health and safety standards in the workplace and the maximum amount of time to be spent at the workplace. However, certain occupational groups, such as doctors, are excluded.

These directives could have a significant impact on the working conditions of health workers in this country. They will provide a minimum standard for all employees and demonstrate the benefits for many workers of belonging to the EU, as the community is now known, following Maastricht. The Maastricht Treaty of 1992 also contained new chapters dealing with the environment, consumer protection and health. There was no mention of health in the Treaty of Rome and prior to 1991 the EC did not possess a formal policy on public health. There is no Directorate-General (DG) for health within the Commission.

COMMUNITY INSTITUTIONS

The European Council

The Council was created in 1974. It is made up of national presidents, prime ministers and foreign ministers. It maps out the strategic direction of policy making in the European Union, especially on contentious issues such as agricultural policy and the budget. These are contentious because of the lobbying undertaken by powerful groups, for example the blockade of French ports by French fishermen. British farmers have also set up pickets following the UK government's decision to ban the sale of beef on the bone (this came into force from 16 December 1997) because of the small risk of contracting Creutzfeldt–Jakob disease (CJD). The Council of the European Union meets twice yearly and may also hold summits if the EU is confronted by a crisis, as illustrated by the growing concern of member states regarding bovine spongiform encephalopathy (BSE) and the sale of beef. The meetings are held in secret. The Labour government, elected in 1997, is committed to making these meetings more open (Dynes & Walker 1995).

The Council of the European Union

The Council is the decision maker of the EU. It is chaired by each member state for 6 months (the presidency) on a rotational basis and is composed of one minister for each member state government and for each subject. Prime minister Tony Blair was president of the Council of the EU from January until June 1998.

There are over 20 different councils with different responsibilities, such as agriculture, foreign affairs, trade and so on. It is the responsibility of the rotating presidency to organize the work of the individual councils, to set priorities and to achieve consensus. The Council examines legislative proposals from the European Commission and amends, accepts or rejects them in conjunction with the European Parliament. It is assisted by a committee of permanent representatives which is made up of the ambassadors of member states to the EU. The committee of permanent representatives usually examines commission proposals in the first instance. If agreement cannot be reached the ministers concerned debate the legislation. Following the Single European Act in 1986 a wide range of issues can now be decided by qualified majority voting. For this each member state has a number of votes, related to the size of its population. The larger countries, including Britain, have 10 votes whereas Luxembourg has only two votes.

The Commission

The Commission is composed of 20 commissioners, nominated by the governments of member states. The larger states nominate two commissioners and the smaller states have one. They are expected to be independent and neutral of their national governments when they are in office. Britain has authority to nominate two commissioners. Traditionally, one is a Conservative and the other a member of the Labour Party. In 1998 they were Nigel Lawson (previously a Conservative MP with experience as a member of Cabinet under Margaret Thatcher's leadership when she was prime minister of the UK) and Neil Kinnock (who was leader of the Labour Party in opposition to Margaret Thatcher). They hold power for 5 years and the term is renewable. The Commission is often described as the 'engine room' of the EU, and it has substantial powers of policy initiation and policy implementation. The Council of the European Union and the European Parliament, however, provide some check on the Commission. The European Parliament has to give its consent to the appointment of the Commission and the European Council appoints the president. It has its own secretariat.

The Commission's work is divided into Directorates-General (DG). There is no DG for health so the lead is usually taken by DG for employment and social affairs (DG V); health and safety issues are also part of the remit of the DG V. Other Directorates-General involved in health matters include DG VIII (development), which has a health and AIDS section, and DG XI (environment, nuclear safety and civil protection). More coordination and consultation is needed to respond to the health chapter in the Maastricht Treaty 1992 (Ludvigsen & Roberts 1996).

The European Parliament

The European Parliament is the only directly elected institution of the EU and elections are held every 5 years. The Parliament was first elected in 1979. In the UK there was an electoral turnout of 32.3% in 1979 and 36% in 1994; this perhaps indicates a low level of interest or awareness of the EU. Electoral turnout in national elections has decreased over this period and so this may just indicate disenchantment with the democratic process (see Ch. 3). The UK has 87 members of the European Parliament (MEPs); their constituencies are made up of approximately 6–7 parliamentary constituencies. In England, Scotland and Wales voting is by the 'first-past-the-post' system, whereas in Northern Ireland, which is one constituency, the three MEPs are elected by the single transferable vote – a form of proportional representation (COI 1994). The British Labour government is committed to extending this proportional voting system for all European elections (Labour Party 1997). The powers of the European Parliament have gradually been extended since the Single European Act 1986, and the Maastricht Treaty on European union 1992. Before then, it was seen as little more than a talking shop and an advisory body. The European Parliament's approval must be obtained before the Council of the EU adopts a legislative proposal from the European Commission; and the European Parliament's assent is needed for decisions on the accession of new member states. The European Parliament has to approve the budget.

MEPs are divided into 20 standing committees. One of the largest is the committee on the environment, public health and consumer protection. This committee has been concerned with the distribution, classification, labelling and advertising of pharmaceutical products; the labelling and advertising of tobacco products; food policy; and the Europe Against Cancer campaign. The Europe Against Cancer programme 1987–1989 was the first major disease prevention programme undertaken by the EU, but other programmes have followed, such as smoking in public places and Europe against AIDS 1996–2000 (Ludvigsen & Roberts 1996). The European Commission has given financial assistance to the European Public Policy Network on AIDS. Individuals have the right to lobby their MEP. Information about the European Parliament and the work of the EU is available from local and university libraries (some useful addresses are included at the end of this chapter).

The European Court of Justice

Under the Treaty of Rome 1957 the European Court of Justice was established to ensure that community law was correctly interpreted and implemented. It is the supreme court of the European Union. The court has fifteen judges, one from each member state, who serve for a 6-year term. The court is based in Luxembourg. The European Court of Justice adjudicates on EU law and a significant body of case law has now been established. All courts in Britain have to take notice of the European Court of Justice. One of the main functions of the court is to give rulings on cases referred to it by national courts. An example of this was the Marshall judgement of the European Court of Justice, 1986. Miss Marshall worked as a senior dietician for Southampton and South East area health authority (AHA) between 1966 and 1980. The AHA's written policy in relation to retirement was that in general female employees should retire at 60 and male employees at 65. Miss Marshall was allowed to continue working until 62 when she was dismissed. She complained to an industrial tribunal that she had been unlawfully discriminated against, contrary to the Sex Discrimination Act 1975 and European law, based on the Equal Treatment Directive of 1976. Eventually, the case reached the court of appeal, who sought a preliminary ruling from the European Court of Justice on the issue of EEC law. The court affirmed that the Equal Treatment Directive had direct effect in the UK, despite the lack of UK legislation that should have been established to implement the directive. As a result of this judgement, retirement policies have been changed in the National Health Service and women may continue to work until 65, if they wish (Marango 1986).

THE EU AND NURSING

When the UK became a member of the EEC, one of the first effects on nursing was a change in pre-registration training programmes. In June 1977 two nursing directives were agreed by the member states. The first directive (77/452/EEC) was concerned with the mutual recognition of diplomas, certificates and other evidence of the formal qualifications of nurses responsible for general care. This was to facilitate the movement of nurses within the EC, 'freedom' being one of the basic rights of individuals living in the EC. The second directive (77/453/EEC) concerned the minimum standards of professional training of nurses responsible for general care. This directive stipulated the length of courses (a minimum of 4600 hours), the subjects to be studied, and the clinical instruction required. These changes were included in the Nurses, Midwives and Health Visitor Rules (1983), a statutory instrument in the UK, which came into effect on 1 July 1983. This directive was revised in 1991 following advice from the advisory committee on training in nursing (ACTN) which advises the European Commission. The ratio between theoretical and clinical instruction was formalized and the directive stipulated that the length of theoretical instruction should amount to not less than one-third and that of clinical instruction to no less than one-half of the minimum length of training of 4600 hours (89/595/EEC). (This was originally a Council of Europe agreement – Strasbourg, 1978.)

Other directives, including health and safety, new laws on maternity leave, and a European code of conduct on sexual harassment, also affect nurses.

Standing committee of nurses of the European Community

The standing committee of nurses of the European Community was established in 1971. It brings together national nurses' associations from all the member states and is the official liaison committee for nursing. The Royal College of Nursing represents the UK. It provides a broad platform for developing policy and practice and for influencing European decision making on all areas which affect nursing, including working conditions and the delivery of health care. The UKCC and the National Boards have consolidated links with other organizations within the EU, particularly in relation to nurse education.

OTHER ORGANIZATIONS IN EUROPE

Council of Europe

The Council of Europe was founded in 1949, before the EC, and now has 32 full member countries and 10 countries with observer status. Britain was a co-founder with 19 other nations. The Council of Europe is dedicated to parliamentary democracy and has three main activities:

- inter-governmental cooperation

- judicial work of its Commission and the Court of Human Rights in Strasbourg

- debates in, and recommendations from its parliamentary assembly.

In 1949, Britain signed the European Convention on Human Rights, which had been drafted by British lawyers, and is administered by the European Commission on Human Rights. Britain, as discussed earlier, has no written constitution and no written Bill of Rights for its citizens. In other countries, citizens seeking protection under the Convention have their cases dealt with in their own country first. British citizens have to apply to Strasbourg. The number of cases doubled in the 1980s. People who are mentally ill, prisoners and immigrants have used this process (Jones et al 1991). The Labour government has made a commitment that the European Convention on Human Rights will be incorporated into British law.

World Health Organization

The World Health Organization (WHO) was founded in 1948 and is a specialized agency of the United Nations, with primary responsibility for international health matters and public health. The WHO has six regional offices, with one for Europe based in Copenhagen, Denmark, which has a nursing and midwifery unit. The European region has over 40 member states.

The WHO convened the first European Conference on Nursing in 1988 in Vienna. It was agreed that nursing practice should be based on the primary health care approach set out in the Declaration of Alma-Ata 1978; innovative nursing services should be developed to focus on health rather than disease. The next phase in the nursing programme of the European regional office was to set up the 'Nursing in Action' project based on a 6-year plan. The project concentrated on two main areas: nursing leadership and practice, and the development of nursing practice. The WHO can help nurses to share experiences and prevent duplication of effort. The nursing and midwifery unit is establishing a database of projects on good practice, in partnership with the European network of WHO collaborating centres for nursing.

In her summary of the seven booklets produced by the Health For All nursing series, Salvage (1993) stated that three universal theses appear to influence the development of nursing in every country:

1. Lack of power. In no country of the region do nurses play a full part in policy making and decision making at all levels of the health care system.

2. Gender. In every country women make up the vast majority of the nursing workforce. They share characteristics of female dominated professions, that is low status, lack of recognition and low pay.

3. Medicalization. Medicine dominates every health care system and acute medical treatment receives prestige and resources.

The WHO, through their position statements and political influence, provide guidance and ideas. Their expertise can be used to address and resolve problems and generate models of good practice. The WHO is also active in the field of patients' rights in regard to quality of service.

EUROPE AND LINKS WITH THE HOUSES OF PARLIAMENT

Arrangements have been made in both Houses of Parliament to keep members informed of EU developments and to enable members to scrutinize and debate proposals for EU legislation and other policies before they are approved by the Council of Ministers. Although the government has agreed not to approve proposals until they have been debated in Parliament, the qualified majority voting system has undermined this agreement. Both Houses of Parliament have select committees that scrutinize European legislation. It has been suggested that such scrutiny could best be exercised by transferring the proposals to the select committee responsible for the policy area in question (as described earlier). Greater cooperation could perhaps result from MEPs becoming members of parliamentary committees, because of their greater knowledge and access to information about the legislative proposals (Dynes & Walker 1995).

CONCLUSION

This chapter has examined role and function of Parliament and the EU. The UK's membership of the EU has had an impact on the UK's constitution and policy making process. Nurses and nursing have also been affected by membership of the EU, predominantly in relation to the rights of employees, the elimination of discrimination in the labour market and the form and content of nurse education. As we have demonstrated, nurses and the patients that nurses care for are all affected in many ways by national and European health and social policies. However, most nurses have paid little attention to Parliament and the EU. Nevertheless, these institutions affect nurses' daily work and the education practitioners receive, and control what practitioners can and cannot do. An understanding of these institutions is essential if nurses are to influence the policy making process.

■ **QUESTIONS FOR DISCUSSION**

- Should tobacco sponsorship be banned in the UK and EU?
- What are the health implications if no advertising ban is imposed?

(cont'd)

■ **QUESTIONS FOR DISCUSSION** (*cont'd*)

- Will sovereignty in the UK be eroded with the advent of Scottish and Welsh devolution?
- Will closer integration with Europe result in a higher standard of education for nurses and more career opportunities?

RECOMMENDED LISTENING

On Sunday evenings, from 22.00 hrs to 23.00 hrs, there is a radio programme on Radio 4 called 'Westminster hour'.

USEFUL ADDRESSES

The European Commission has offices in the UK:

8 Storey's Gate, LONDON SW1P 3AT. Telephone: 0171 973 1992

9 Alva Street, EDINBURGH EH2 4PH. Telephone: 0131 225 2058

4 Cathedral Road, PO Box 15, CARDIFF CR1 9SG. Telephone: 01222 371 631

9/15 Bedford Street, BELFAST BT2 7EG. Telephone: 01232 240 708

REFERENCES

Birch A H 1993 The British system of government, 9th edn. Routledge, London

Clay T 1987 Nurses, power and politics. Heinemann, London

Central Office of Information 1994 Parliament, 2nd edn. HMSO, London

Dearlove J, Saunders P 1991 Introduction to British politics, 2nd edn. Polity Press, Cambridge

Department of Health 1989 Working for patients. HMSO, London

Department of Health 1992 The health of the nation: a strategy for health in England. HMSO, London

Department of Health 1998 Our healthier nation: a contract for health. HMSO, London

Dynes M, Walker D 1995 The new British state. Times Books, London

Hart C 1994 Behind the mask: nurses, their unions and nursing policy. Baillière Tindall, London

Jones B, Gray A, Kavanagh D, Moran M, Norton P, Seldon A 1991 Politics UK. Harvester Wheatsheaf, New York

Jones M, Gough P 1997 Nurse prescribing – why has it taken so long? Nursing Standard 11(20):39–42

Labour Party 1997 New Labour because Britain deserves better. Labour Party, London

Ludvigsen C, Roberts K 1996 Health care policies and Europe: the implications for practice. Butterworth Heinemann, Oxford

Marango R 1986 The retirement age of health visitors and school nurses. Health Visitor 59(5):160

Salvage J 1993 Nursing in action: strengthening nursing and midwifery to support Health for All. WHO Regional Publications, European Series 48. WHO Regional Office for Europe, Copenhagen

Wise M, Gibb G 1993 Single market to social Europe. Longman, Harlow

Wolff J 1996 An introduction to political philosophy. Oxford University Press, Oxford

Power, politics and nursing

Sian Maslin-Prothero and Abigail Masterson

■ **CONTENTS**

INTRODUCTION

The traditional study of politics concentrated on the state and the various institutions of government such as Parliament and the judiciary. However, the prevailing contemporary view is that politics occurs whenever there are differentials in power; that is any social relationship which involves differentials in power is political. Nursing and health care are clearly political issues as scarce resources are allocated amongst competing and arguably equally worthy groups and needs. Even the development of nursing knowledge has a political aspect to it. For example nursing theorists and researchers must be accepted by the wider

scientific community and be thinking in a politically acceptable way if they are to have their work taken seriously.

Nurses need to influence the political agenda in order to
challenge the current inequitable access to health and health
care resources, economic impoverishment and unsafe physical surroundings which threaten the health and well-being
of countless people in the UK. An understanding of power
is central to this quest, but as Cohen (1992, p. 113) states: 'the
concept of power is one that has been too long overlooked
by nursing educators, authors, theorists and researchers'.
Gilbert (1995) asks how can we claim to be empowering
others when we have no notion of what power is.

Power and the politics of nursing are therefore the focus of
this final chapter. We develop further the theme of power
that has underpinned the previous discussion of the importance of politics and its impact on the profession of nursing,
the context of care and the content of practice. Through this
final analysis we hope to encourage nurses to respond in an
informed way to present and future challenges confronting
the profession.

Nurses currently work in health care systems that exclude
or disadvantage large numbers of people who need care and
they are frequently confronted by health problems caused
by ageism, sexism, racism and the inequitable distribution
of resources. In addition, the consequences of environmental neglect and devastation threaten health on a global scale.
Despite explicit commitments to health promotion by the
profession, nurses tend to focus on patients/clients as individuals and on the minutiae of the nurse–patient relationship rather than the macro sociopolitical context of health
and health care. Consequently nurses rarely challenge the
structures within which they work and tend not to address

fundamental issues such as inequality that may determine health status, and which permeate health care structures and can constrain nurses' ability to deliver health care. Nurses can bring about change in health and social policy and, arguably, this is our professional responsibility. For example, our statutory body, the United Kingdom Central Council for Nurses, Midwives and Health Visitors, states in the Code of Conduct that: 'Each registered nurse, midwife and health visitor shall act, at all times, in such a manner as to: safeguard and promote the interests of individual patients and clients; serve the interests of society' (UKCC 1992, p. 1).

In order to achieve this change in perspective and mode of practice nurses need to understand power and how it operates (both overtly and covertly) to shape the construction of health and illness, the provision of health care and the structures within which that health care is provided. The ability to challenge the marginalization and subordination of the nursing voice in current political debates is dependent on this knowledge. That is, power cannot be tackled and harnessed unless it is recognized and understood.

To this end, we begin by exploring the concept of power and introducing key theoretical perspectives on the operation of power in social systems.

DEFINITIONS OF POWER

Power is one of the most evocative words in the English language. It frequently conjures up images of coercion and domination (Farrier 1993). All too often it evokes negative feelings among nurses. Nevertheless, power pervades all aspects of life and nurses must begin to understand and use it if they are to succeed in achieving their organizational goals. Political theorists have spent many years attempting to define power and explain its impact. Defining power is not easy because it has so many different meanings and connotations depending on the context in which it is being used. For example it can be viewed as both a positive and negative force. There have also been many attempts to describe the nature of power and to differentiate it from authority, domination and influence. The most general meaning of power is simply ability, and power in the political sense is usually taken to mean the ability to make other people do what you want them to do (Raphael 1976). Within the policy arena, power refers to the process by which the values and interests of one group are acted upon over and above the values and interests of another. Foucault (1983) argued that competition for resources leads to differential power relations as particular groups achieve access to and control of resources through exerting control over weaker groups. These power relations are then secured by the parallel emergence of a discourse that promotes these social relations as 'natural'. Lukes (1974, p. 24) maintains similarly that power concerns the complex and subtle ways in which institutions serve to shape people's cognitions, perceptions and preferences so that they 'accept their role in the existing order of things, either because they can see or imagine no alternative to it, or because they see it as natural and unchangeable, or because they value it as divinely obtained and beneficial'.

Freire (1972) saw oppression as being derived from the ability of the dominant group to establish their values and norms as the 'right ones' and to use this power to enforce them. He saw the process of oppression as beginning with the entrenchment of the values position of the dominant group and the internalizing of those values by the subordinate group in the belief that this will bring to them the same power and control held by the dominant group. Exposing distorted power relations is the basis for emancipatory and empowering work.

In health care, the medical model, which impacts on the nature and composition of health services in all care settings, has been of fundamental importance to the maintenance of the power of the doctors. For example student nurses learn to think and act in ways which are defined for them by the dominant group within the health system – that is doctors – and which they accept as natural commonsense views of reality.

THEORIES OF POWER

We now introduce three classic perspectives on power and consider their application to nursing. These perspectives by no means comprise the full extent of the power literature but serve to provide a useful introduction to key thinking in this area.

 Steven Lukes (1974) classified these perspectives as the three faces of power. They have also been referred to as the dimensions of power. It is important to note that these theories, because of their complex nature, have been very difficult to research and demonstrate empirically.

One-dimensional power

The primary exponent of pluralism, Robert Dahl (1961), suggested that in order to determine who held power in any situation conflict had to be observed and the outcome of actual decisions had to be examined. In this way the individual or group who held power would be revealed. From this perspective the individuals or groups whose preferences prevail in conflicts over key political issues are seen to be the ones who exercise power in the political system (Ham & Hill 1984).

The second level of power

This view of power was criticized by Bachrach & Baratz as being too simplistic (1962, cited in Dearlove & Saunders 1984). Bachrach & Baratz developed the idea of a second level of power which operated covertly by suppressing conflicts before they occurred and thus prevented issues from entering the political process. This was known as 'non-decision-making'. According to Bachrach & Baratz, power not only involved the ability to shape the outcomes of decisions but also the ability to dominate the political process so that some issues never arise and certain decisions never get made, in order to protect the status quo. They argued, therefore, that if only the process of decision making is studied the power involved in preventing issues from emerging would not be identified. Bachrach & Baratz suggested three ways in which a powerful élite may stifle issues from entering the political system: firstly by ignoring political demands so a decision one way or another is not necessary; secondly by ensuring awkward political demands are never raised, by encouraging disadvantaged or less powerful groups to think that there is no alternative or that change is impossible; finally by preventing people from formulating grievances in a coherent way, through control of the media, schooling and shaping of preferences through socialization.

Three-dimensional power

In this theory power is seen to be located not so much in

individuals or groups of people, as in the two perspectives above, but instead is manifest in what Dearlove & Saunders (1984) referred to as systems of domination. In this way power relationships penetrate the very structures of society itself. Lukes (1974) argued that from this perspective power involves the shaping of people's preferences so that neither overt nor covert conflict exists. Power relationships have become routinized and, as Dearlove & Saunders (1984, p. ii) explain: 'involve(s) sets of social relations in which one party has established routine command over another, such that he or she is rarely challenged'.

Rules with unequal outcomes are obeyed as a matter of course without conflict. Power is accepted as a 'normal' part of relations that exist between certain groups in different social settings, spheres of activity or policy making and implementing. This explanation supports the notion of institutionalized inequalities – that is inequalities occurring at a systemic level and underpinned by ideologies such as sexism, racism or ageism, for example. Here institutional rules, procedures and practices generate unequal outcomes, regardless of the motives of individuals involved. In other words the system is biased, not individual behaviour (Dearlove & Saunders 1984). A system of domination, therefore, is socially constituted behaviour in accordance with rules, norms or values, backed by formal or informal sanctions of approval or disapproval and inclusion or exclusion. A system of domination becomes internalized or accepted as part of the natural order of things (Ham & Hill 1984). Lukes (1974) argues that through this process a false or manipulated consensus may exist whereby people's wants are formed by the society in which they live, and these may not be the same as their real needs or interests. Difficulties obviously exist here in determining exactly what people's real or 'unfalse' consensus may be. As Lukes pointed out, this can only be determined by studying what people would choose when expressing choice free from the constraints of their socialization, a situation that is impossible to achieve.

SYSTEMS OF DOMINATION

Critical or social action approaches to social and political analysis which involve exposing such systems of domination have gained increasing attention in the nursing literature as a means of understanding nursing and its relationship to society at macro and micro levels. Oppression within such perspectives is thought to result from the ability of dominant groups to impose their norms and values on society so that they are accepted as the *right* ones, readily enforced because of the power held by the dominant group. The dominant group looks and acts in a way that is different from the group that is being oppressed, resulting in the attributes of the subordinate group being devalued. The norms and values of the oppressor are internalized by the oppressed, who believe that the only way to achieve power is to mimic the characteristics of the oppressor. Overcoming oppression is believed to start with recognition or consciousness raising.

NURSES AS AN OPPRESSED GROUP

It is important to note at this point that nurses are not a homogenous group. Nursing has several ancestries that represent competing values and ideals. For example the gentle, angelic, selfless woman epitomized in many portrayals of Florence Nightingale and the militant trade unionism which emerged from the asylums and poor law institutions (Owens & Glennester 1990). Nursing is also split into subgroups by specialty and place of work: 'What counts as nursing may vary a lot, and sometimes even nurses find it difficult at first to recognise that what other nurses are doing is really nursing' (RCN 1992, p. 18). Similar barriers exist between and within practitioners, educators, researchers and managers. Each group possesses different values and these values are often in conflict with one another (White 1984, Cooke 1993). Because of the imbalance of power between practitioners, educators, researchers and managers, in many cases these groups have not been united in their pursuit of common goals. The barriers of specialty, heritage, grade and perhaps even gender have frequently prevented the profession from speaking with one voice. We defend our portrayal of nurses as an oppressed group by the evidence interspersed throughout this book that nurses lack autonomy, accountability and control over their working environments and the scope of their practice. We also acknowledge that this powerlessness may well be linked with the social oppression of women generally. Since the end of the 19th century there has been a drive for professionalization in nursing, which has increased in intensity since the 1970s in the UK. This commitment to changing the status of nursing has been articulated vociferously in the professional press and was encouraged by the establishment of degree courses in nursing. Both the early reformers associated with the drive for registration and the contemporary reformers demanding better education and an evidence base for the profession have adopted strategies pioneered by the doctors before them (Davies 1995, Rafferty 1996). However, the traditional model of professionalization sought by such groups is, of course, a gendered one organized around male patterns of career development and priorities.

Nurses have been lambasted by many commentators because nurses have seen being political as inappropriate.

However, the situation is far more complex than it appears. For example, in the fight for registration in the early 20th century nurses marshalled political and social power effectively to meet their ends (see Ch. 6). Similarly there were nurses within the women's suffrage movement. Throughout our more recent history nurses working in mental health and learning disabilities, who were mainly men of course, have fought successfully for power both within and without the profession. It is within general nursing that the non-political attitude has seemed strongest. There seems to be a fear that becoming political will damage the caring ethic, stability and respectability of nursing. For example, Alison Dunn, in the foreword to Jane Salvage's seminal text on the *Politics of nursing* (Salvage 1985) wrote: 'Many nurses are uncomfortable with the word "politics". It belongs to a world which they do not feel, nor want to be part of. Politics is for others. Politics is a deviant activity in which no self-respecting professional should indulge.'

In the 1997 general election two nurses, Ann Keen and Laura Moffat, were returned as Labour MPs. Increasingly too nurses are playing a role in local government, for example Linda East, one of the contributors to this book. Without wishing to exert too much pressure on these particular individuals it should be interesting to see whether this makes any difference to the profile of nursing within key policy making institutions and to the aspirations of nurses about how they can make a difference and promote the health of the population.

It appears that despite significant moves towards greater sexual and racial equality and the development of the supposed classless society, health care environments continue to be class dominated and racist and patriarchal in nature (Sweet & Norman 1995, Gough & Maslin-Prothero 1994).

The nurse–doctor relationship is seen by many to replicate patriarchal and class relationships in wider society. Thus female nurses take on a subordinate role in the male-dominated medical division of labour. Care work itself is seen as a natural extension of the female role and therefore perceived to be less privileged in status than cure work. Nurses are more likely to be drawn from the working or middle classes, whereas doctors tend to be upper class. Stein's (1967) classic work on the doctor–nurse game is a good example of coercive power relations in action. Stein illustrated the doctor's traditional responsibility for making decisions regarding patient management and detailed the complex process through which nurses recommend actions without challenging the doctor's control, thus maintaining the status quo. He argued that the rules of the doctor–nurse game require that nurses can only make recommendations about care in such a way that the idea appears to be initiated by the doctor. In his view such power relations were upheld and reinforced by the complex socialization process embedded in medical and nursing training. Later work by Stein, Watts and Howell (1990) suggests rather encouragingly that nurses were increasingly being recognized by their multidisciplinary colleagues, the media and the public as advanced practitioners with independent duties and responsibilities to their patients and clients. Stein et al attribute much of this changed perception to the move of nursing into higher education. The higher education environment, coupled with a view within much of nursing academia that doctors are narrowly focused technicians who merely treat illness, is thought to have encouraged student nurses to believe they are equal to other health care providers. However, a series of short but extremely critical comments on nursing in the British Medical Journal (Short 1995), headlined '*Has nursing lost its way?*' and calling for a return to the old nursing values, suggest the power and pervasiveness of the medical agenda on nursing in the UK. We would be unlikely to see the work of medicine and doctors discussed in such an authoritative and possessive way in a nursing journal. Similarly, few other professional groups undergo the intense media scrutiny on their mode of dress and titles as nursing.

Another example of coercive power relations in nursing and health care is to be found in the situation of black people who are well represented in the NHS as nurses but usually found in the lower grades and less popular specialties. During the 1950s and 1960s selection committees set up in Commonwealth countries recruited people to work in the health services (King's Fund 1990). Many of the recruits were directed towards enrolled nurse training and to what were perceived to be less prestigious areas of nursing such as the care of older people and people with mental health problems or learning disabilities (Baxter 1988). The Commission for Racial Equality (1992) has suggested that some NHS managers believe that the presence of significant numbers of black nurses in the NHS is evidence that the NHS is not a racist institution. However, it is clear that black people have little opportunity for promotion and therefore little influence over the shape and structure of service provision. There is evidence that the number of black people applying for nurse education is falling despite an increase in the number of black 18-year-olds in the population. Baxter (1988) suggests that this may be because family and friends who currently work in health care are actively discouraging them as a result of their own experiences of racism and discrimination.

The power of managerialism and medicine combined has had a significant impact on the shape of nursing for the next century. Increasingly, nursing work is becoming more specialized along disease-related parameters. For example specialist nurses are being employed to care for patients/clients with particular medical conditions such as epilepsy, Parkinson's disease and so on.

Managerialism and its associated focus on efficiency, effectiveness and value for money has increased the division of nursing tasks on the basis of skill mix. Patient-focused projects and the re-engineering of health services have drawn attention to the need to restrict the use of expensive nursing resources for complex tasks challenging the holistic total care approaches predominant in the profession's 'New Nursing' discourse, which prevailed in the mid-1980s. In fact, many would argue that the doctor's handmaiden appears to have been reborn as a consequence, in the so-called nurse practitioner and advanced practice roles which are gaining more popularity in the 1990s. Such nurses appear to be becoming more medical, taking on the role(s) formally undertaken by junior doctors. The preparation and training for such roles and the management of post-holders are often controlled by medicine and management rather than nursing. The ease with which this has been achieved can be partially explained using Lukes's third face of power, explored above – nurses have internalized the values of medicine in the hope that by becoming mini-doctors and attaining the characteristics of the powerful they too can become powerful (Harden 1996).

And yet, despite all this 'good' behaviour, nurses continue to be undervalued in comparison to doctors and managers when it comes to pay (Buchan, cited by Day 1996). As we write, the unions representing nurses have announced their demand for a pay rise of up to 20%, to compensate for the way nursing pay rates have fallen behind those of other professions and to prevent nurses from leaving the profession

(Radio 4 1997). Hart (1994) notes that doctors, although often full of praise for nurses, rarely make any effort to alter the balance of power between nursing and medical staff. In fact attempts at nursing innovation or independence, such as the pioneering nursing development unit on Beeson Ward in Oxford, have often been thwarted as a result of medical intervention.

Midwives have steadily been reclaiming the ground lost in the medicalization of childbirth, chronicled so ably by Oakley and others (see for example Oakley 1984, O'Sullivan 1987). Their central role as independent providers of care has been recognized within the 'Changing Childbirth' initiative. However, Littler (1996, p. 29) reflects on an opportunity she had of joining: 'a group of high flying GPs in a fast-growing health centre ... and become their own midwife'. The chance of leaving the hierarchical hospital management was tempting, but eventually not tempting enough. She felt that GPs are reluctant to share the decisions, power and burden with other health care professionals in the practice (i.e. nurses, midwives and health visitors), and she felt that too much energy would have been spent on exerting her rights, rather than enhancing her practice as a midwife. McCoppin & Gardner (1994) note that the ability to exercise political power depends not only on sheer numbers but also on having a strategic position in the workplace such that other workers cannot be used as substitute labour. In addition, McCoppin & Gardner argue that power depends on group characteristics that are not easy for nurses to acquire; that is, predominantly male composition and membership of the upper social classes.

NURSES AS OPPRESSORS

Within the British health care system of the 1980s and 1990s there has been an increasing emphasis on individuals taking responsibility for their own health and illness, and a feeling that a harmful dependency has been fostered by the state provision of universal welfare.

Through the empowerment of patients and clients, nurses believe that people (and groups) can seek to alter repressive relationships. We have a dichotomy here. On the one hand we are attempting to be powerful and create change. But we are also trying to empower our patients and clients while, at the same time, trying to develop our own power base. Hart (1994) argues that the notion of empowering service users necessarily means taking power from someone else. Mulholland (1995) asserts that in their haste to rally to the rhetoric of the empowerment discourse, nurses have failed to examine critically the socioeconomic and political dynamics of nurse–client relations. Nurses and midwives are still viewed by users, with justification, as having all the power, no matter how disempowered nurses themselves feel.

An example of this is the effect of the Mental Health (Patients in the Community) Act 1996. This Act gives the 'supervisor' (often a mental health nurse) the legal power to identify where the client lives, gain access to the client and the power to take the client (against his/her will) to a place of treatment, employment or education. As Rogers (1996, p. 9) argues: 'The community mental health nurse takes on, in effect, the custodial role of yesteryear's asylum attendant'.

Nurses claim to be the advocates of patients and yet patients are dependent on them for care. Patients are reluctant to challenge decisions made about their care for fear of being labelled difficult. The introduction of the *Patient's charter* (Department of Health 1991) encouraged patients to expect and demand certain things from health care providers. Copies of the *Patient's charter* were delivered to every household in England and Wales, and yet many users either remain ignorant of their rights or are unable to exert them.

As Price & Mullarkey (1996, p. 16) state, when clients are referred to mental health services the nurse is often in a position of power. Yet within the therapeutic counselling relationship there should be 'a dynamic of power-sharing, with one or other party being more powerful at different stages in the relationship'.

Hewison's (1995) observational study of nurses' interactions with patients showed how nurses use language as a means of exerting power and controlling patients in the clinical environment. Nurses give the impression of communication and collaboration with clients and patients, but often, on closer examination, control is the key.

EDUCATION AND POWER

This section will argue the case for power and politics as a legitimate part of nursing knowledge and will also explore developments in nurse education as a means of illustrating political power in action. Rafferty (1996:1) reminds us that 'education lies at the centre of professional work and expertise and therefore occupies a pivotal position in the shaping of occupational culture and the politics of nursing'.

Nursing has been heavily dependent on medicine for its knowledge base and focus of practice. When nurses began undertaking courses in higher education establishments and studied disciplines such as physiology, psychology and sociology, their introduction to the ideas and methods of inquiry advocated by such disciplines began to exert their influence on the development of nursing knowledge. It is only recently, therefore, that social policy and politics have been included in nursing curricula and deemed a suitable and even valuable knowledge base for nurses to study. For example nurse educators at what was the Avon and Gloucestershire College of Health (now the University of the West of England) describe the importance of empowering student nurses by giving them the tools to examine the organizational context within which they work. The resulting module, for which they won a King's Fund partnership award in 1994, was entitled *Power, policy and practice* and explored the concepts of power in relation to nursing (Aust et al 1997). Purposeful reflection on the nature and structures of power and oppression, as offered by this course, is suggested by many political theorists as being crucial to emancipation and action. Latterly, however, there appears to have been rather a backlash against the social content of many curricula. Critics in the health service have bemoaned an apparent clinical skills deficit of nurses on qualification and a lack of biomedical and pharmacological knowledge. Educationalists have felt pressured to reduce the focus on the broader social science base in curricula and increase the amount of biological sciences taught. Students are receiving more skills training and being introduced to the acute care environment earlier.

Glen (1990) argued that nurse teachers must address power relations both within higher education and between nursing and the wider social and political domain which influences and constrains them. Certainly, the move into higher education of nursing education provides an illuminating illustration of the complexity of power and systems of domination at macro and micro levels. At least to begin with, the move was seen as an empowering one and evidence of societal recognition of the value of nursing and the developed state of nursing knowledge. Yet nurses may find themselves marginalized, devalued or in conflict with other health professionals (James & Field 1996, p. 73). This can be explained by the different educational approaches taken in the past.

Doctors and the professions allied to medicine have long been educated in higher education settings, while nurses were formerly constrained in apprenticeship-style training. However, the move to more diploma and degree courses for pre- and post-registration nurses and increased shared learning between professional groups, optimists argued, should result in an increased knowledge base for nurses and may well, in time, alter the power relationships between the different health care professionals. For example commentators who had attributed nursing's political invisibility in part to a lack of confidence forecast rapid change as nursing students enjoyed the benefits of a university education rather than a vocational training apprenticeship. Learning alongside medical students, they argued, would help destroy the mystique of medical knowledge and power and nursing would maintain professional control of the curriculum with less dependence on service demands.

Unfortunately the reality has been rather different. In many instances nursing students are university students in name only, frequently being taught in isolation on dedicated campuses far from their seat of learning. Nursing education has often been located in the 'new' universities away from medicine, which has remained in the older universities, so opportunities for shared learning remain limited. Nurse educators themselves have found marrying the expectations of the professional bodies with university requirements in the terms of academic levels and assessment expectations traumatic. Nurse educators have been reviled in the academic press, and by many of their new academic colleagues, for their lack of research and publication experience. In addition, the centralization that resulted from the reorganizations led to massive early retirements and redundancies. And despite being located in universities, the development of educational purchasing consortia composed of service representatives has once again increased the control of the service over the shape and content of the education provided. Mulholland (1995, p. 446) points out that: 'The failure of nursing and nurse educationalists to confront power as a feature of their relations with each other and their clients is closely related to their failure to recognise the inextricable relationship between knowledge and power'.

NURSES AS A POLITICAL FORCE

As the contributors have noted time and time again in this book, nurses are 'notoriously bad at being political' (Casey 1996, p. 1), not only regarding their role and place in existing health care structures but also about other issues and areas which affect health. Hanley (1987) suggested those nurses with higher academic levels were more likely to participate in protests, voting, campaigning, etc. If this is the case this could have an interesting impact on nursing and health as the nursing workforce raises its general educational level through increased numbers of diplomates and graduates in the profession.

It has been suggested that leadership is lacking in nursing because the people attracted to nursing, and perhaps specifically recruited to it, tend to be submissive, lacking in initiative and obedient (Harden 1996). For those who seek higher office, exercising leadership involves additional responsibilities including being in a position where power and authority can be used to influence or impact others

(Dean 1995, Henderson 1995). Yet if nurses feel uncomfortable with notions of power and politics it is not surprising that they shy away from assuming leadership skills and responsibilities. Nevertheless, nurses are not a homogenous group as we have already noted – there are a multitude of differing types and levels of nurses from student nurse to nurse manager, as well as a variety of disciplines such as midwives, mental health nurses, health visitors and so on. Each of these groups has its own set of values and priorities and it is important to consider these differences in any analysis.

CONCLUSION

We have argued that a broad understanding of the operation of power within health care institutions and local, national and international politics is of fundamental importance in order for nurses to influence proactively the political agenda for health gain. The lack of political insight and the profession's inability to recognize and manipulate power has contributed to nurses' historic invisibility and powerlessness.

An appreciation of the way power is exercised and the way it operates overtly and covertly through 'systems of domination' is of profound importance to nurses and nursing. The ability to challenge the marginalization and subordination of the nursing voice within policy decision making circles, as well as in the face of medicine, is dependent upon this knowledge. The power dynamic cannot be tackled unless it is known and understood. The overt operation of power, by its very nature, is easily recognized. The covert operation of power is much more difficult to recognize and therefore to change. Also nurses have found it sometimes easier to own up to being the victim of powerful relationships, rather than the perpetrator of subordination within a broader system of professional domination.

Such a large and diverse profession as nursing has faced difficulty in achieving a single voice on many political and professional issues. Policy makers in health care have consistently shown their disregard for nurses. Changes that have major implications for nurses, their work and the patients they care for are imposed upon them with little reference to them, their needs or interests (Hart 1994). Nevertheless, it would be inaccurate to portray nurses as being either totally helpless victims of more powerful groups, or as exploiters of professional control. Rather, nurses and nursing swing from one end of this continuum to another. Nurses must fight back against a persistent lack of professional power, and examine their practice in terms of enabling their clients or patients to make informed choices about their health.

The boundaries between the different health care disciplines and the nature of the structure and funding of health care are fluid rather than fixed and are historically and socially constructed by the complex interplay of power between different groups (Rafferty 1996, p. 191). However, analyses of the type modelled in this text help nurses become aware of the power relations anchored in race, gender and class. Such awareness, we believe, can facilitate the emancipation of nurses from these oppressive social systems in order that nursing and nurses can achieve their full potential for social good.

FURTHER READING

Aust R, Fraher A, Limpinnian M, Maslin-Prothero S, Mowforth G, Miers M, Thomas D, Wilkinson G 1997 Power, policy and practice. University of the West of England, Bristol

This is a resource pack developed by the sociology theme team at what was formerly the Avon and Gloucestershire College of Health after they won the King's Fund nurse education prize for 'Innovation and development in nurse education'. It is copyright free and can be used by nurse educators to introduce nursing students to issues of power policy, and practice.

REFERENCES

Aust R, Fraher A, Limpinnian M et al 1997 Power, policy and practice. University of the West of England, Bristol

Baxter C 1988 The black nurse: an endangered species. National Extension College, Cambridge

Casey N 1996 Editorial. Nursing Standard 11(2):1

Cohen L B 1992 Power and change in healthcare: challenge for nursing. Journal of Nursing Education 31(3):113–116

Commission for Racial Equality 1992 Ethnic minority hospital staff. CRE, London

Cooke H 1993 Boundary work in the nursing curriculum: the case of sociology. Journal of Advanced Nursing 18(12):1990–1998

Dahl R A 1961 Who governs? Yale University Press, New Haven

Davies C 1995 Gender and the professional predicament in nursing. Open University Press, Buckingham

Day M 1996 Two-tier treatment: why pick on us? Nursing Times, 92(8):18

Dean D 1995 Leadership: the hidden dangers. Nursing Standard, 10(12–14):54–55

Dearlove J, Saunders P (1984) Introduction to British politics. Polity Press, Cambridge

Department of Health 1991 The patient's charter. HMSO, London

Farrier B 1993 The use and abuse of power in nursing. Nursing Standard 7(23):33–36

Foucault M 1983 Afterword: the subject and power. In: Dreyfus H L, Rabinow P (eds) Michel Foucault: beyond structuralism and hermeneutics, 2nd edn. University of Chicago Press, Chicago, pp 208–226

Freire P 1972 Pedagogy of the oppressed. Penguin, London

Gilbert T 1995 Nursing: empowerment and the problem of power. Journal of Advanced Nursing 21:865–871

Glen S 1990 Power for nursing education. Journal of Advanced Nursing 15(11):1335–1340

Gough P, Maslin-Prothero S E 1994 Women and policy. In: Gough P, Maslin-Prothero S E, Masterson A (eds) Nursing and social policy: care in context. Butterworth Heinemann, Oxford, pp 135–153

Ham C, Hill M 1984 The policy process in the modern capitalist state. Wheatsheaf Books, Great Britain

Hanley B F 1987 Political participation: how do nurses compare with other professional women? Nurse Economics 5(4):179–188

Harden J 1996 Enlightenment, empowerment and emancipation: the case for critical pedagogy in nurse education. Nurse Education Today 16:32–37

Hart C 1994 Behind the mask: nurses, their unions and nursing policy. Baillière Tindall, London

Henderson M C 1995 Nurse executives: leadership motivation and leadership effectiveness. Journal of Nurse Administration 25(4):45–51

Hewison A 1995 Nurses' power in interactions with patients. Journal of Advanced Nursing 21:75–82

James V, Field D 1996 Who has the power? Some problems and issues affecting the nursing care of dying patients. European Journal of Cancer Care 5:73–80

King's Fund 1990 Racial equality: the nursing profession. Equal Opportunities Task Force, Occasional Paper, No. 6. King's Fund, London

Littler C 1996 Power struggle. Nursing Times 92(31):29

Lukes S 1974 Power: a radical view. Macmillan, London

McCoppin B, Gardner H 1994 Tradition and reality: nursing and politics in Australia. Churchill Livingstone, Melbourne

Mulholland J 1995 Nursing, humanism and transcultural theory: the 'bracketing-out' of reality. Journal of Advanced Nursing 22:442–449

Oakley A 1984 The captured womb: a history of the medical care of women. Blackwell, Oxford

O'Sullivan S (ed) 1987 Women's health: a Spare Rib reader. Pandora Press, London

Owens P, Glennester H 1990 Nursing in conflict. Macmillan, Basingstoke

Phillimore P, Beattie A, Townsend P 1994 Widening inequality in health in Northern England, 1981–91. British Medical Journal 308:1125–1128

Price V, Mullarkey K 1996 Use and misuse of power in the psycho-therapeutic relationship. Mental Health Nursing 16(1):16–17

Radio 4 1997 Today programme. 12 September 1997

Rafferty A M 1996 The politics of nursing knowledge. Routledge, London

Raphael D D 1976 Problems of political philosophy, 2nd edn. Macmillan, London

Rogers B 1996 Supervised discharge: implications for practice. Mental Health Nursing 16(2):8–10

Royal College of Nursing 1992 The value of nursing. RCN, London

Salvage J 1985 The politics of nursing. Heinemann, London

Salvage J 1992 The New Nursing: empowering patients or empowering nurses? In: Robinson J, Gray A, Elkan R (eds) Policy issues in nursing. Open University Press, Milton Keynes, pp 9–23

Short J A (1995) Has nursing lost its way? Dual perspective, British Medical Journal 311(7000):303–305

Stein L I 1967 The nurse–doctor game. Archives of General Psychiatry 16:699–703

Stein L I, Watts D T, Howell T 1990 The doctor–nurse game revisited. New England Journal of Medicine 322(8):546–549

Sweet S J, Norman I J 1995 The nurse–doctor relationship: a selective literature review. Journal of Advanced Nursing 22:165–170

UKCC 1992 Code of professional conduct. UKCC, London

White R 1984 Nursing: past trends, future policies. Journal of Advanced Nursing 9:505–512

Glossary

Agenda 21
Agenda 21 was established at the 'Earth Summit' of 1992, where world governments met to discuss the global environment, which resulted in the global action plan for sustainable development. Agenda 21 calls on local authorities throughout the world to develop their own 'Local Agenda 21', i.e. a local action plan for sustainable development.

Back-bencher
A member of parliament without portfolio.

Cabinet
A committee of the principal members of the British government such as the secretary of state for health. The Cabinet is chaired by the prime minister. The prime minister determines the Cabinet agenda, decides how issues will be dealt with, can announce the decision of Cabinet without taking a vote and makes Cabinet appointments.

Collectivism
A political-economic theory that argues that the means of production and/or distribution should be collectively owned or controlled, or both, and not left to the actions of individuals pursuing their self-interest. Socialism and communism are collective ideologies and promote the desirability of public ownership in the interests of the community as a whole. This collective ownership can include state property and cooperative institutions. The owners (the public) have varying degrees of control.

Constitution
The established form of government in a kingdom or state. This may

be a written document, as in the USA, or unwritten, as in the UK. Constitutions set out the powers of the various organs of government and the standards for determining the legality of their actions. Constitutional change usually results from judicial review.

Corporatism
A revival of the theory of the corporate state popular in the 1920s and 1930s. Developments in the 1960s and 1970s in all Western societies suggested that public decision making was increasingly becoming a tripartite affair of bargaining between the state, employers' associations and trade unions. In return for a share in the making of political decisions, the non-state organizations were expected to be able to discipline their members and to deliver them in support of the agreed policies. In the 1970s the failure of the TUC to control its member unions and the inability of the unions to control their own members led to its rejection.

Democracy
The form of government in which the sovereign power is in the hands of the people, and exercised by them directly or indirectly. Derives from the Greek meaning the rule of the *demos*, or the citizen body. The size of modern nation states has meant that (apart from those that include provision for referenda in their constitutions) democracy is no longer direct but indirect, i.e. through the election of representatives, hence the term representative democracy.

Devolution
Transfer or delegation of authority from central to regional government.

Efficiency
A managerial and political concept associated with value for money. Efficiency is concerned with getting the best relationship between inputs and outputs. In the context of health care this has led to extending the hours of use of expensive capital equipment such as MRI scanners and reviewing skill-mix in clinical environments.

Empowerment
To enable.

Equity
Justice or fairness.

Fascism
Fascism was a product of the deep-seated social and economic crisis in Europe following the First World War. It produced no coherent system of ideas and the various fascist movements reflect the very different national backgrounds of the countries in which they developed. None the less there were some common traits. All were strongly nationalist, violently anti-communist and anti-Marxist. All hated liberalism, democracy and parliamentary parties, which they sought to replace by a new authoritarian state in which there would be only one party, their own, with a monopoly of power. Racism and anti-Semitism were features of some fascist movements, such as that in Germany in the years before the Second World War.

Feminism
A social and political philosophy and movement which supports the claims of women to social, political and economic equality with men.

First-past-the-post
An electoral system where the candidate who receives the largest number of votes is the person elected. The first-past-the-post system is used in the UK.

Franchise
The right to vote.

Free market
A market which is not impeded by any form of government intervention.

Front-bench
The foremost bench in either Parliament (that is the House of Lords and House of Commons) assigned to either ministers or ex-ministers.

Green Paper
A consultative document where a government sets out proposals for discussion, for example the Department of Health (1998) *Our healthier nation* Green Paper.

Ideology
Political or social philosophy. Set of values and beliefs.

Laissez-faire
The principle of non-interference especially by government in industrial and commercial affairs.

Liberalism
A political philosophy which values individual freedoms. Liberty is of great importance and includes the right to free speech, religious practice and intellectual and artistic expression. State activity is restricted to the maintenance of law and order, the defence of the realm and to safeguard the conditions in which commerce and trade can flourish.

Marxism
The theory that human and political motives are at root economic, and that the class struggle explains the events of history. The state is seen to function in the interests of capitalism and therefore in the interests of the owners of the means of production rather than the workers.

New Right
The New Right is a political ideology which is committed to the free market and to the restraint of public expenditure. New Right proponents, for example Margaret Thatcher, sought to reduce the state's involvement in all areas of economic and social life.

Patriarchy
The term patriarchy is derived from the Greek 'rule of the father' and describes the authority and control exercised by men over women.

Pluralism
Pluralism refers to a view of society where there is no dominant political, ideological or cultural group. No one interest group is dominant in the policy process, instead there is balance and fair competition.

Quasi-markets
A term coined to describe the operation of free market principles to

state institutions. For example the purchaser/provider split in health care established a quasi or 'as if' market in state funded health care.

Racism
A belief in the superiority of one race over another.

Select committee
Members of parliament specially chosen to examine a particular question and report on it to parliament. The constitution of select committees represents the division of seats along party lines in the Houses of Parliament.

Sovereignty
Sovereignty means the possession of ultimate legal authority on decision making. Eurosceptics argue that the powers of the European Parliament are undermining the UK government's sovereignty over domestic policy. In the UK the sovereign is the monarch, that is the Queen, who is the head of state.

Statutory instrument
An amendment to existing legislation.

Suffrage
The right to vote, especially in parliamentary elections.

Welfare
Government support for the poor, particularly the free or subsidized supply of certain services, for example health care and education.

White Paper
Statement of government policy intentions. The White Papers *Working for patients* and *Caring for people*, published in 1989, introduced the Conservative government's plans for reforming the NHS which were formalized in the NHS and Community Care Act 1990.

Index